# Childhood Psychosis in the First Four Years of Life

# Childhood Psychosis in the First Four Years of Life

HENRY N. MASSIE, M.D.
JUDITH ROSENTHAL, M.S.W.

McGRAW-HILL BOOK COMPANY

New York • St. Louis • San Francisco
Auckland • Bogotá • Hamburg • Johannesburg • London • Madrid
Mexico • Montreal • New Delhi • Panama • Paris • São Paulo
Singapore • Sydney • Tokyo • Toronto

Library of Congress Cataloging in Publication Data

Massie, Henry N.
  Childhood psychosis in the first four years of
life.

  Includes bibliographical references and index.
  1. Psychoses in children.  2. Infant psychiatry.
I. Rosenthal, Judith.  II. Title.  [DNLM: 1. Child
development disorders.  2. Psychotic disorders—In
infancy and childhood. WS 350 M417e]
RJ506.P69M37  1984        618.92′89        83-26799
ISBN 0-07-040765-7

1234567890    DOC/DOC    8987654


ISBN 0-07-040765-7

The editors for this book were Thomas H. Quinn and Michael Hennelly,
the designer was Christopher Simon, and the production
supervisor was Reiko F. Okamura. It was set in Baskerville
by Achorn Graphics, Inc.
Printed and bound by R. R. Donnelley & Sons.

*To Our Families*

# Contents

# Acknowledgments

B. Kay Campbell, Ph.D., now with the Division of Family Medicine, Wayne State University School of Medicine, Detroit, co-developed the Scale of Mother-Infant Attachment Indicators During Stress. And Kenneth Wulff, M.D. of Hayward, California joined us for the Piagetian-based cognitive study of the children. In addition along the way, many other colleagues have assisted generously with their skill and patience—Margaret Lock, Candace Pearce, Eleanor Willemsen, Riva Nelson, Martha Harris, Joel Saldinger, Marguerite Van Remoortere, Kathy Bacon, Mark Sullivan, Abbot Bronstein, Robert Zachary, and Gloria Hirsch. Mimi Horne has been our fine illustrator. Several teachers have given us invaluable guidance—Justin Call, Eleanor Galenson, Joe Afterman, Al Scheflen, Calvin Settlage, and Phil Spielman. We also share a special bond of knowledge with our patients who joined us for sometimes difficult journeys. Lastly, the L. J. and Mary C. Skaggs Foundation, the Morris Stulsaft Foundation, the Carl Gellert Foundation, Childrens Hospital, San Francisco, and St. Mary's Hospital, San Francisco, all gave needed support to make this work possible.

## Credits

Versions of chapters 6 and 8 appeared respectively in the *Journal of the American Academy of Child Psychiatry,* Vol. 17, 1978, and the *Journal of Autism and Developmental Disorders,* Vol. 10, 1980. Parts of Chapter 6 also originally appeared in *Child Psychiatry and Human Development,* Vol. 7, 1977, pp. 211–230.

The *Scale of Mother-Infant Attachment Indicators During Stress* formerly appeared as a chapter in *Frontiers of Infant Psychiatry,* edited by J. Call, E. Galenson, and R. Tyson, Basic Books, 1983.

# Childhood Psychosis
# in the First Four Years of Life

# Introduction

The study of childhood psychosis has been a stepchild to the investigation of adult schizophrenia. Chronologically, systematic research began decades after work on adult psychotic illness; nosologically, for years children were classified in terms borrowed from the lexicon of adult illness; and most significantly, psychiatrists and psychologists attempted to understand major emotional illness in children on the basis of existing models for grown-ups, or to see it as some special category or subcategory of the more familiar and socially troublesome adult psychoses. Thus until relatively recently, the study of adult schizophrenia was hypothetically adapted to fit the special case of children. This historical tendency, however, may have been a tragic example of putting the cart before the horse. Whatever it was, it greatly slowed progress in the field. For we are only relatively recently beginning to study the childhood psychoses from a developmental perspective in which a child's psychobiologic maturation from conception is scrutinized carefully for clues to what has gone wrong. This approach also gives new life to the study of adult psychosis, for it is possible that the developmental defects discovered in children may be the same as or similar to those contributing to psychotic breakdowns in later life.

Shakespeare—a brilliant clinician schooled only in life—recognized the primacy of childhood when he evoked the "seven ages" of man, and when he had Hamlet utter, "They say an old man is twice a child." Likewise, Freud's epic unravelling of the nature of adult neuroses began with his delineation of the contribution of infantile sexuality (1905) and its vicissitudes to subsequent complexes and conflicts, all arrived at through introspection, observation of children, and reconstructions from the psychoanalysis of adults.

This volume describes our own as well as others' research that starts very close to the beginning of life. Our own study, *The Early Natural History of Childhood Psychosis Project,* uses *films of the infancy of children prior to diagnosis of a childhood psychosis.* These movies function as prospective data gathered retrospectively from parents who had made home movies of their children in infancy before they became ill. Produced in this normal fashion, the films provide visual information about the first year of life in children who subsequently became ill which has been unavailable heretofore. Our study couples these films with clinical data to focus on the very early life of a number of children who suffer from the major psychotic conditions of early childhood: autism, symbiotic psychosis of childhood, childhood schizophrenia, and mixed form of early childhood psychosis. The ultimate distinctiveness of these syndromes from each other, and even from adult schizophrenia, is neither clear nor proven. Yet at the same time, in some areas, relatively discrete syndrome profiles appear to emerge from our own and others' work that lead us toward empirical divisions. With the data from our cases, we have sought to identify problems in mother-infant social interaction and bonding, and to link these to the failures in intrapsychic structuralization of the child and to symptomatology. That is, we have tried to understand how a group of children translate certain external events into internal experiences which profoundly compromise their growth.

We integrate our own identification of early social behaviors and understanding of psychological structuralization in the very young child with a significant part of contemporary research in child psychiatry and child development. This mode attempts to specify particular maturational failures in a disturbed child (whether organic or psychological); to connect them with the particular stage at which a function should have developed; and to identify what may have been an internal or external traumatic interference at that stage and at that time in the child's life. The data which our research has provided is predominantly psychological—growing from the histories and therapies of the children and families—and social-interactional, growing from the analysis of filmed behavior. Therefore, the theory-building is largely on this level: that is, it is integrated with psychoanalytic developmentalist postulates as to the nature of the mental development of the young child, although it is also integrated with current biologically oriented research in this area. Ultimately, we have aimed in this volume to synthesize the findings of The Early Natural History of Childhood Psychosis Project with other strands of developmental research in such a way that knowledge of the traumatic influences and developmental failures which underlie psychotic illnesses becomes more precise.

To do this we have organized our presentation first to provide multidisciplinary material as a backdrop against which to view our own study. In Chapter 1, we review the history of investigation into the childhood psychoses. Chapter 2 reviews past diagnostic nomenclature and advocates a basic nomenclature for syndromes of early childhood psychosis for clinical and research use, a nomenclature which we use consistently throughout the book. Chapters 3 and 4 review contemporary research in normal child development which relates to our own study and methodology of looking closely at early mother-infant social behavior and the process of psychic structuralization of the infant. Chapter 5, which begins our report of The Early Natural History of Childhood Psychosis Project, delineates the methodology of our own studies. Following this, Chapter 6 provides ten clinical case studies from the Project. Chapters 7 and 8 report empirical studies of the early attachment behaviors of the infants and mothers in the Project compared with a matched group of normal mothers and infants, along with a Piagetian-based study of the cognitive development of the subjects and the matched normal children. In Chapter 9 we review and summarize the findings of the Project studies. Chapter 10 integrates the findings of abnormal development with understanding of the normal process of early psychological maturation so as to revise and refine aspects of the theory of causation of childhood psychosis. Chapter 11 incorporates the evidence the Project has provided on the emotional, social-interactional, and cognitive deficits of the severely ill young children into principles of treatment of children suffering an early childhood psychosis who come to therapy in the first four years of life. The Appendix contains the Scale of Mother-Infant Attachment Indicators During Stress (ADS scale). This scale focuses on the process of parent-infant attachment behaviors—gazing, touching, holding, affect, vocalization, and proximity—and is a clinical instrument, derived from the Project findings, for use by pediatricians and infant-care workers in the service of early identification and treatment of disturbed parent-infant dyads.

An underlying theme throughout is the Project's attempt to make more concrete the definition, meaning, and mechanism of the damage of such phenomena as parental overprotectiveness, nonprotectiveness, coldness, remoteness, overstimulation, rejection, hostility, and anxiety. In doing this, in general, the basic unit of our focus is the mother-child dyad. By "mother," however, we mean the child's principal caretaker, who might also be a surrogate parent or a father. But in almost all instances the principal parent has been the natural mother, although for the sake of variety we use the terms "parent," "mother," and "caretaker" interchangeably. We focus on the mother-infant dyadic process because of its fundamental importance to child development, yet, as the case histories reveal, this unit exists in a complex context where grandparents, husbands, social custom, economics, and so many other influences all buffet or support the mother and her baby. They all bring forth the next generation.

We cannot and dare not predict what will happen in any given family, the influences are so many and so subtle. But when we do recognize that something is going wrong—that there is depression, apathy, or chaotic aggression in a parent or infant—we must try to invervene in an ameliorating way. This is the task of our work: to identify as early as possible symptoms of emotional illness and the behaviors that are causing them, and to prevent their crystallization into stubborn, grim illnesses.

# Chapter 1

# Historical Background

Throughout the history of psychiatry, relatively little has been written on the subject of the psychoses of childhood compared to the abundant child-psychiatric literature in other areas. In 1880, Maudsley, perhaps aware of the reason for this, wrote "How unnatural! is an exclamation of pained surprise which some of the more striking instances of insanity in young children are apt to provoke" (quoted in Kanner, 1971, p. 14). He was recognizing the intense aversion people have to seeing and responding to the troubling and bizarre behavior of children suffering a psychotic illness; where there should be promise of life, there is instead emotional stunting. Even professionals tend to shy away from the disease because, in addition to the children's eccentricity, the symptomatology is not easily understandable or treatable.

It is therefore useful to begin with an account of how physicians have thought about psychotic illness in children over time—from its first dismissal as a global, incomprehensible condition of "lunacy" to the many subsequent careful attempts to make it more understandable and therefore treatable. This small aspect of the history of psychiatric medicine describes the establishment of childhood psychosis as a legitimate subspeciality of child psychiatry. To be more precise, this chapter recounts the identification, classification, and study of childhood psychosis as a psychiatric subspecialty. With the study of any childhood psychopathology, the problem always arises of distinguishing actual disease from normal developmental immaturity. Keeping this in mind, it is the highly bizarre behavior and the long-lasting break with reality that in general distinguish the childhood psychoses from other forms of childhood psychopathology as well as from simple developmental immaturity.

To examine the roots of the study of childhood psychosis, we must follow the historical line of development of child psychiatry proper as it grew out of adult psychiatry and pediatrics. From the vantage point of descriptive medical history, we shall survey the early documentation of cases which appeared to be forms of childhood psychosis, along with their rudimentary classifications and explanations. In this century, research in childhood psychosis has become less influenced by work on adult schizophrenia, and pioneering efforts have been made to carefully delineate subtypes, classificatory systems, etiological theories, and treatment modalities. The syndromes of childhood psychosis became a field for innovative work from all of the different theoretical perspectives of psychiatry. Only recently, with increased knowledge of child development, are we able to study childhood psychosis from a developmental perspective which scrutinizes psychobiologic maturation from birth for clues as to what has gone wrong when illness occurs.

## "Prehistory"

Before the twentieth century, however, there was what Walk (1964) has termed a "prehistorical" period in child psychiatry. Walk reviews the early pediatric literature for descriptions of epilepsy and sleep disorders which may be among the first real accounts of mental disorders in children. He quotes Ruhrah's *Pediatrics of the Past* and Still's *History of Pediatrics,* written at the end of the fifteenth century, on cases of sleep disorders, nightmares, bedwetting, and convulsions which contemporary texts might more accurately place in the domain of child psychiatry. Further, Walk cites a sixteenth-century Alsatian, Oesterreicher, as the first to mention psychological disturbances of children as having psychogenic causes. For this physician, good mental habits in children could be corrupted by what they saw and heard, even by music. A sixteenth-century Italian pediatrician, Mercurialis, perceived environmental causes of stammering, and advocated treatment by "driving out an emotion, usually fear" at the root of the trouble.

In the seventeenth century, Brouzet wrote on infantile jealousy and rivalry. An infant may "pine" because of jealousy, and even though very young, can show rivalry. Here he went against the grain of his time in which children, let alone infants, did not impress people as having developed emotions. But with unusual thoughtfulness, Brouzet advised parents to give enough attention to the jealous infant, but in such a way that the rival older child would not suffer.

In the eighteenth century a series of interesting reports were written throughout Europe. In Amsterdam, children afflicted by epidemics of mass hysteria fell down in violent convulsions that lasted up to an hour. Diagnosed as being possessed by the devil, they received exorcisms which had the effect of bringing on further somatopsychic symptoms and episodes. For example, they vomited nails, rags, and other foreign bodies that they had secretly swallowed.

In the mid-eighteenth century, Greding described a child as born "raving mad." Witnesses claimed that when the infant was four days old it took four women to hold him down; he tore everything near him, climbed onto furniture, and had "fits of uncontrollable laughter."

In 1770, Prefect described the case of an eleven-year-old patient. For four months, he kept daily journals of the boy's course. In these he speculates as to the etiology of the prolonged confusional states and restless delirium which alternated at times with stupor or despondency. Prefect eliminated possible causes when he felt them lacking in evidence; he found no defective brain tissue, no hereditary predisposition, and no worms. Further, the child had not been traumatized by fright or punishment. While he did not describe the nature of the treatment, if any, Prefect describes a complete recovery in four months. The significance of this case historically is the precision of the clinical detail, both in terms of the symptomatology of the illness and of the mobilization of available knowledge for consideration of etiological factors.

Haslam (1799) records three cases of children seen at the Bethlehem Institution who, close to puberty, had the onset of an illness descriptive of simple schizophrenia. Burrows (1828) reports a twelve-year-old boy with choreiform movements and speech impairment who died after six years. Significant for his attempt to differentiate organicity and retardation from functional nervous illness, Burrows felt that if the child had been suffering the latter, his illness would have appeared after puberty. He reasoned that defects in intellect were the primary etiological agent of mental illness: younger children, he thought, were not sufficiently developed intellectually to have a nervous disease, but they could be retarded, since that was but a manifestation of organicity.

Rush, the pioneering American psychiatric physician, made the earliest direct acknowledgment of psychosis in childhood in a discussion of "insanity in children" in his first psychiatry textbook in 1812. Observing four disturbed children, two of whom were pre-pubescent, he inferred that "madness" equated with biting their mothers and themselves, and he attributed their behavior to an "unsteady" condition of their brains, which were susceptible to transient mental impressions. He also believed that the neurological immaturity of the children would not allow for a permanent state of insanity, but that healthy developmental processes would take over and the condition would abate. It is noteworthy, despite the questionable conclusions he reached, that Rush brought developmentally oriented thinking to bear upon theory.

In Paris, Voisin (1826) observed institutionalized children, and divided them on the basis of their symptomatology and speculated etiology into four categories: (1) the feeble minded, with intellect between idiocy and normal; (2) those born normal, who had had faulty education; (3) those showing character abnormalities from birth, such as pride or uncontrolled "passions"; and (4) those born of insane parents who were thereby genetically disposed to mental illness. Voisin developed a treatment which consisted of enlarging the child's intellectual sphere, improving interpersonal relationships, and providing moral education that aimed at suppressing antisocial tendencies.

When lack of money forced Viosin to close his institution, he joined the staff at the children's annex of Bicêtre. This facility was exclusively for retarded children. Here he worked with Seguin (1846), who advocated that the retarded could be therapeutically restored to a relatively normal life outside the institution. This was progressive thinking for a century which viewed retardation as a hopeless condition, and Seguin polemicized against well-known physicians of the time, one of whom was Esquirol. Esquirol himself (1838) described several mentally ill children between the ages of eight and eleven; and he drew for the first time a clear distinction between dementia and idiocy, reserving idiocy for severe congenital defects. The distinction clarified prognosis, for, he believed, recovery was only possible in dementia because its symptoms could be suppressed. Nonetheless, Seguin, in his turn, refused to accept that idiots, or retardates, had a poorer prognosis; he claimed that with proper treatment, they could be restored to a socially adaptable level of functioning. And a major outcome of Seguin's work was the establishment of treatment centers for retardates throughout Europe.

Two striking single case studies appeared in the mid-nineteenth century. Morrison, in 1848, described a six-year-old girl with convulsions and inflammation of the brain who subsequently became violent, incoherent, and antisocial. He noted her sudden recovery after a year of institutionalization, but without speculating on why she improved. The second case study was MacDonald's, in 1846, of a boy who at four years became excited when his parents refused him an outing. They punished him severely, and following this he went into paroxysms of terror, became violent, and passed into a state of stupor. He recovered in six months. Like Morrison's case, the description was vivid and detailed, but no attempt was made to use it to create a framework out of the meager literature on childhood mental illness of the time.

In 1867, Maudsley included a chapter on "insanity of early life" in the first edition of his pioneering British psychiatric text. He tried to correlate symptoms he had observed with the developmental status of the child, suggesting a system of seven categories: monomanias, choreic mania, cataleptoid insanity, epileptoid insanity, mania, melancholia, and affective insanity. Despite the limitations of the nosology in terms of inclusiveness and applicability, it was the first such system put forth. Maudsley had also taken the developmental immaturity of the child into account. But his efforts were not appreciated by his colleagues; they harshly criticized him "for daring to acknowledge the existence of insanity in children." Nonetheless, childhood psychosis relatively soon afterward became a legitimate topic of enquiry, and Kanner believes Maudsley's text to be a landmark in the history of the study of the illness. Ironically, the subsequent literature on childhood psychosis rarely cites Maudsley.

In 1883 two researchers posited organic etiological models of childhood psychosis. Cleavinger (1883) attributed cases of insanity in children to their unstable nervous systems. He also believed these severe disturbed conditions to be "larvated" epilepsies. At the time, Cleavinger compiled a review of the world literature on mental illness in children: it contained fifty-five references. Spitzka, in the same year, suggested a model in which a genetic substrate rendered a child vulnerable neurologically to nutritional deficits. Like Maudsley, he took the immaturity of the child into account, and stated that true insanity was rare in children because development would rectify mental functioning in most instances. Spitzka theorized that delusions, primary symptoms of true psychosis, required for their formation the more advanced cognitive apparatus of adults. Spitzka's work is noteworthy historically for the amount of attention he gave childhood psychosis in his text, *The Treatment of Insanity*. In addition to his basic genetic-organic model, he speculated on the etiological significance of various environmental factors, such as fright, sudden changes in temperature, and masturbation.

Other literature at this time picks up on the environmental etiological models and adds a psychological component signifying a swing of the historical pendulum away from the organic viewpoint, a swing that would see further reversals in the future. Kerlin (1879) wrote that insanity was more common in children than previously believed and that its development was related to the child's experiencing traumatic situations earlier in life. While not specifying the nature of the trauma, he believed that the very young child could either recover or later manifest dementia, criminal tendencies, and other serious behavioral disorders. Kerlin was before his time in pointing to the effects of nonphysical trauma on a child's later development of ego deficits.

By 1883 Alexander was considering the psychological and developmental aspects of normal children in order to understand abnormal children. As a consequence, he found that families where illness arose in children seemed to have more tortured and troubled histories than the families of normal children. In 1894 Taylor elaborated on possible psychological and environmental causes. He hypothesized that precocity, fright, punitive religious teaching, superstition, brutal parenting, and long periods of deprivation and exposure could lead to severe emotional disturbances in children.

Thus, these early attempts in the nineteenth century to understand the basic causes of insanity in children predestined the more sophisticated specialized conceptualizations of the twentieth century. Rubenstein's (1948) scholarly review of the literature on childhood psychosis in America in the nineteenth century recognizes the growing interest in the illness during the last decade of that century, interest which foreshadowed the search for more precise etiological models and the abandonment of the lexicon of "insanity in childhood" and "childhood lunacy" for the description of more specific syndromes such as "infantile autism," "childhood schizophrenia," and "symbiotic psychosis of childhood."

Several significant trends emerge in the survey of the field of childhood mental disorders from the first reported cases in the sixteenth century through the end of the nineteenth century. There was increasing systematization of the descriptions of the symptomatology; and, while the samples were small, increasing attempts were made to delineate retardation from mental illness. There were scholarly attempts to distinguish organic from psychological etiological factors. Further, there was increasing effort to take the neurological and psychological immaturity of the child into account. Thus, prior to the twentieth century we have a series of phenomenological accounts of severe aberrations of mental functioning in childhood and adolescence.

## The Twentieth Century

With the twentieth century, descriptive elaboration continues, and the study of adult psychosis reasserts an influence on the study of childhood psychosis in both positive and problematic ways. Child psychiatry proper also comes into being, with childhood psychosis as a subfield. The rest of this chapter considers the influence of modern adult psychiatric study of schizophrenia on child psychiatry, and continues the survey of the investigation of profound childhood mental illnesses in the areas of etiology, differential diagnosis, and treatment.

In the next few decades, the work of Kraeplin (1896/1919) and Bleuler (1911/1950) in adult psychiatry had great significance for childhood psychosis. In 1896 Kraeplin presented his final formulation of dementia praecox in the Fifth Edition of his *Textbook of Psychiatry*. He introduced a new nomenclature for adult psychosis, teasing out specific syndromes of catatonia, hebephrenia, simple deterioration, and paranoia which previously had been gathered under the broad category of dementia praecox. Kraeplin's work was organically based; he proposed the cause of dementia praecox to be either metabolic or central nervous system degeneration.

Following Kraeplin's terminology, child psychiatry's history for the next two decades was largely the study of dementias of childhood. Noteworthy were DeSanctis' (1906) work on dementia praecocissima and Heller's (1908) on dementia infantalis. Studying institutionalized children, DeSanctis claimed that the "decline" in psychotic children was not deterioration, but a reversible regression. Thus his important contribution was twofold—the introduction of the concept of regression and the clear distinction between severe emotional disturbance and retardation in children. In his turn, in 1908 the Austrian educator Heller reported six cases of an infantile mental illness which he felt took an unusual course. The onset was in the third or fourth year of life after prior normal development. The symptoms were an increasing malaise, rapid diminution of interests, loss of language function, and loss of sphincter and other motor control. Heller's disease was regarded as the earliest form or manifestation of dementia praecox, and therefore a functional psychosis.

Bleuler's *Textbook of Psychiatry* in 1911 initiates two changes in nomenclature. First, the term "schizophrenia" superseded dementia praecox. Second, in accord with Kraeplin's division of the illness into syndromes, Bleuler stated that there is not one schizophrenia but a multiplicity of conditions, hence the "group of schizophrenias." Bleuler disagreed with the Kraeplinian view that deterioration was inevitable, and he placed more emphasis on the psychological features of the psychotic manifestations—understanding them as having both defensive and adaptive functions, an extremely important clinical insight. In addition, he added further specificity by positing his famous "four A's" for diagnosis of schizophrenia: affective disturbance, autistic withdrawal from external reality, ambivalence, and association (or thought) disorder. These fundamental findings are present to some extent in every schizophrenic patient. There are also variable accessory symptoms, termed secondary symptoms, such as hallucinations, delusions, and psychomotor distortions.

Bleuler surpassed Kraeplin in his attempt to give psychotic symptoms a mental function or content and a psychological structure. In doing this, he was influenced by the then-developing Freudian theory. Still, the central focus of Bleuler's understanding of schizophrenia was the underlying thought disorder that was present in all cases, whether latent or manifest.

Following Bleuler's use, the term "childhood schizophrenia" began to appear in child psychiatry. Earlier in the first decade of the twentieth century, Kraeplin's influence had replaced the vague terms of "lunacy," "insanity," and "madness" with the more precise "dementia infantalis" and "dementia praecococissima." Then, in 1919, the American psychologist Witmer, in an interesting case history, became the first to refer to profound childhood breaks with reality as "childhood psychosis," in order to distinguish the illness from adult parallels. Witmer (1919) further posited an interpersonal etiological model for the illness in detailing the successful treatment of a 5-year-old boy.

In a study of the "functional psychoses of childhood," Kasinin and Kaufman (1929) reported on all cases over a three-year period at the Boston Psychopathic Hospital. They found only six cases of childhood schizophrenia and concluded that the illness was rare. By contrast, in 1932, Richmond, at St. Elizabeths Hospital in Washington, D.C., asserted how often children diagnosed as mental defectives or retardates may be schizophrenics.

In 1933 Potter described six cases of schizophrenia in children, noting their superficial resemblance to mentally defective children. Potter's criteria for childhood schizophrenia limited the diagnosis to prepubertal children. The major features were: a generalized retraction of interests from the environment; disturbances of thought as manifested by blocking, condensation, perseveration, and incoherence; disorders in language function and sometimes the presence of mutism; diminution, rigidity, and distortion of affect; excessive or inhibited motility, sometimes to the point of immobility; bizarre mannerisms, with a tendency to perseveration or stereotypy. In terms of etiology, Potter speculated that the mothers of childhood schizophrenics were "dominant and overprotective" and the fathers "submissive." Historically, his etiological observations are noteworthy because they are the first specifically to link the illness in the child with character pathology in the parents and particular combinations of parental personality traits. Such thinking forms the basis of many contemporary family interactional and dynamic models of the etiology of schizophrenia.

By the middle of the 1930s, childhood schizophrenia was recognized as a disease entity in the now established field of child psychiatry. Although observers of children had, at first, adopted the nosologic structure of adult schizophrenia in toto, they gradually perceived how child patients displayed dissimilarities in onset of illness and clinical course. Independently of each other, Homburger in Germany, Ssucherewa in Russia, Lutz in Switzerland, and Despert in the United States recognized two syndromes—children whose illness had an insidious onset and those with acute onset.

Despert (1938) added a third group—insidious onset followed by acute fulmination. In agreement with Potter, Despert felt that a child's immaturity modified the usual symptoms of adult schizophrenia. And in agreement with Lutz (1937) she found that hallucinations occurred only after six years of age. One of Despert's major contributions was her study of cognitive processes, especially language function, in childhood schizophrenics. She noted "the child has a capacity above normal to retain words and use them in a mechanical way, although his vocabulary for expression of needs was small" (1938, p. 367). She related this language disorder, and concomitant autistic thinking, to the failure of the schizophrenic child to achieve normal emotional relatedness. And in a further elaboration of the symptomatology of the language disorder, she noted the schizophrenic child's anomalous speech: a dissociation between language, sign, and function; echolalia; and most importantly, how the children do not use language to *communicate meaning.*

Bradley (1941), with a sample of fourteen schizophrenic children and one hundred twenty-four normal control children, found eight behavioral characteristics which distinguished the control from the index group: seclusiveness, irritability when seclusiveness was disturbed, day-dreaming, bizarre behavior, diminution in number of personal interests, regressive nature of personal interests, sensitivity to comment and criticism, and physical inactivity.

Geleerd (1946) noted the high frequency of temper tantrums in schizophrenic children, and she described them as later editions of the small infant's earlier affectomotor panic states. During tantrums, the schizophrenic children were out of contact with reality and acted delusionally as if they were warding off an attacker. She concluded that these children have not established an image of the mother within themselves and consequently are dependent on the actual presence of their mothers; they cannot separate from the parent without withdrawing into an omnipotent fantasy world.

Kanner, the major figure in the study of psychotic children alluded to earlier, in 1943 delineated the syndrome "early infantile autism" from the more inclusive group of childhood schizophrenics. In a series of eleven cases, he demonstrated a grouping of clinical features that he termed "a pure culture sample of inborn autistic disturbance of affective contact." The striking feature was the inability of the children to relate themselves in ordinary ways to people and things from the beginning of life. The "extreme aloneness" of the children from so early in life distinguishes autism from childhood schizophrenia in terms of object relations, for the schizophrenics experienced "withdrawal from formerly existing participation." It remains unclear, however, as to whether Kanner felt that an autistic's isolation began at birth or in the first year of life. Other characteristics noted by Kanner were that the children never molded to their parents when held, they failed to use language for communication, they showed an anxious desire for the maintenance of sameness and a fear of new patterns, and they had a fascination with objects which they could handle with excellent fine motor coordination.

In 1949 Kanner distinguished a subtype of autism in which the children develop normally for eighteen to twenty months of life, then withdraw, lose language, halt social development, and curtail normal activities. He termed this subtype of autism developing in the second year of life "secondary autism," and felt that such children could not be differentiated after the development of the symptomatology from those with early infantile autism.

By 1953, when Kanner had accumulated a sample of one hundred autistic children, he was more inclined to the view that mental illness was largely absent in the childrens' families. And subsequently, he felt that the diagnosis of autism was being applied too loosely to a heterogeneous group of severely impaired children. Fish and Ritvo (1979) ascribed this problem to clinicians' overemphasis of the symptoms of withdrawal and stereotypy, which permitted the inclusion of many severely retarded children with organic brain disorders under the rubric of autism.

While Kanner looked for the maturational sources of illness in the newly described syndrome of autism, Bender emerged as the pioneer in elaborating the search for the inborn or organic factors in the psychoses of early childhood. According to Bender (1947, 1955), childhood schizophrenia involves a maturational lag at the perinatal level which is characterized by a "primitive plasticity" in all areas from which subsequent behavior develops. The child's muscle tone does not respond like that of normal children to stimulation, although he may be hypersensitive to stimuli, and his postural and motor behavior retains immature features. In the youngest children there is a disturbance in homeostatic equilibrium—especially evident because this is one of the major areas of infantile behavior—which appears immature, embryonic, fluid, and unpatterned. From these underlying physiological deficits, Bender postulates that such children have difficulty inhibiting the wish to act on impulses, and that perceptual deficits adversely affect the child's capacity to form social relationships. Thus, immaturity impairs socialization which further contributes to immature behavior and symptomatology. She attributed the extreme anxiety of the disturbed children to their inability to control incoming stimuli. She also described the schizophrenic child's difficulty in forming a body image and psychologically separating the inside of the body from the outside. Bender most often felt that there was a genetic cause for these psychophysiologic and neuropsychological manifestations.

In regard to age of onset, Bender discussed three critical periods (1947): (1) The first three years of life, when the precursors of schizophrenia, in her terminology, appeared, formed the first such period. In these children, development was uneven from birth, and at no point had the child developed normally. (2) The second period was from ages three to four-and-a-half. These children had normal development until this time, and then a regression, either insidious and slow or very acute. Once regressed, the child might slowly regain some patterned behavior and ego functions, but would return distorted by the schizophrenic patterning. (3) The third critical time was prepuberty, from approximately ten to eleven-and-a-half years. Clinically these children were quite different. They regressed in specific areas, and their symptomatology appeared to be more differentiated than syndromes appearing earlier in life. In common with the second group, the prepubertal children also suffered extreme diffuse anxiety.

To recapitulate, Bender theorized that childhood schizophrenia involves a total integrative failure. The diagnosis subsumes many varieties or subtypes, according to her, of which autism is but one. However, in spite of her formidable contribution, her work had its limitations. Her theories were exceedingly complex, involving neurophysiology, psychodynamics, and genetics, and some workers felt that they unnecessarily confused diagnosis. And many of her neurological signs were at the same level of specificity as the "soft signs" described for the vague entity Minimal Brain Damage in the 1960s and 1970s, and its counterpart in the 1980s, Attention Deficit Disorder. These neurological signs are neither indicative of a known central nervous system lesion nor pathognomonic for mental illness.

## The Psychoanalytic-Psychodynamic Tradition

A. Weil (1953) follows Bender's emphasis on the failure of the child to establish balanced homeostatic patterns. In her experience, schizophrenic children have abundant developmental deviations and a history of overintense or underintense reactions from earliest infancy.

She differentiates a special group of severe ego development disturbances that are characterized by a lack of progression as contrasted
with even more serious types of regressive disturbances. Weil defines
the faulty ego as deficient in the development of object relationships,
unable to test or accept reality, and deficient in synthetic function and
use of age-adequate defenses.

Conceptualizations in terms of object relations and the ego's ability
to construct reality and synthetically mobilize defense mechanisms
demonstrate the growing influence of psychoanalytic theory. Since
the 1940s, psychoanalytically informed physicians have progressively
elucidated the failures of psychological development in young
psychotic children and connected them to the often traumatic vicissitudes of the children's relationship with their parents. Bettelheim,
perhaps, takes the extreme position in this tradition, espousing the
view, with vivid case studies (1967), that autism and childhood schizophrenia need not have any organic contribution and that it is the
outcome of severe disturbances in the parent-child relationship. However, clinicians and researchers in the psychodynamic, psychoanalytic
school more typically posit a physical vulnerability or unusual sensitivity (Bergman & Escalona, 1949)—be it on a constitutional, genetic,
perinatal traumatic, neurologic, or biochemical basis—to the untoward nurturing insults which their work describes. Rank and
McNaughton, for example, detailed (1950) the development of a
three-year-old girl they termed an "atypical child." With respect to
her psychologic structures, she did not develop an ego sufficient to
distinguish between herself and the outside world, and she had
marked distortions in libidinal and aggressive drive development.
Symptomatically, she had severe temper tantrums, bizarre posturing,
no conversational speech, and no relatedness to people. They linked
the developmental failure to the chronic overwhelming deprivation,
with but rare instinctual gratifications, that she had suffered. The
child had spent her first months in the hospital because of prematur-
ity, and subsequently was minimally cared for by her mother. Consequently, the nascent ego, unable to mediate between the self and the
external world, was arrested and fragmented.

In this tradition, Mahler and her associates (1949, 1952, 1955)
meaningfully differentiated the syndromes of childhood psychosis on
the basis of the child's failure to achieve specific intrapsychic structures in infancy. Her research methodology—observation of children
in normal and therapeutic nurseries and study of the therapeutic
process with severely disturbed children—outlined the syndrome

which she termed "symbiotic psychosis of childhood" and distinguished it from autism. Thus in autism, according to Mahler, *the baby seems never to have recognized the mother as a representative of the outside world* and never to have emotionally cathected (attached to) her as a separate entity. By contrast, in symbiotic psychosis of childhood the baby does develop a clear early mother-infant relationship; however, further progress to the stage of object libidinal cathexis of the mother does not occur, and the mental representation of the mother is not differentiated from the self. In the symbiotic illness, symptoms (terrors; regression in toileting, feeding, speech, and motility; and self- and other-directed aggression) become apparent in the toddler stage when the normal maturation of the ego and physical capacities lead the child to separate physically from the mother. By contrast, in autism symptoms of lack of awareness and response to the mother may be evident from the first weeks of life.

Mahler conceptualized pathology within the maturational schema of separation and individuation which she and her associates have also outlined from their studies with both normal and ill children (1968). Further, the symptoms also may have a defensive function: autistic withdrawal or fixation may be the way children hallucinate away disturbing perceptions, particularly those that normally elicit an affectionate or angry emotional response. And the symbiotic maintenance of the undifferentiated self-object tie with the mother may be the child's delusional attempt to maintain or restore a parasitic oneness with the mother and ward off catastrophic ego disintegrating separation anxiety. Etiologically, Mahler felt that the determinants were severe and painful illnesses early in life; constitutionally vulnerable or oversensitive infants; and early mothering that was overstimulating, overprotective, very anxious, or remote and nonprotective. The interaction of these factors could interfere with baby's fusion, blending, and separation of good and bad images of people (animate objects) and the self. Instead, confused and distorted fusions of part images of the self and objects develop, and these impair orientation to and perception of reality.

Many other astute clinical investigators have also advanced our knowledge of childhood psychosis in important ways by conveying the bizarre internal reality of psychotic youngsters in terms which share a common ground with Mahler and Rank. Chief among them are Erikson (1950), Bonnard (1967), and Ekstein and Caruth (1969). Szurek and his colleagues (1956, 1973), among others, have also drawn on longitudinal experience with large numbers of children treated over extended periods in the hospital to assert that childhood psychosis is psychogenically rather than organically based; in brief, they feel that "the psychotic child manifests in his disorder the incorporation of and identification with the disorder of both his parents' personalities" (1956, p. 522) and their anxiety.

Contemporaneously, but in a descriptive rather than psychodynamic vein, Creak (1961) collaborated with a group of British psychiatrists in formulating "nine points" for the diagnosis of the "schizophrenic syndrome" in childhood. They drew from the symptoms described by both Kanner and Bender, but at the same time did not mention disturbances of thought which consequently makes their symptomatology applicable to younger rather than older children. The nine points of the British Working Party were: (1) gross and sustained impairment of emotional relationships with people; (2) apparent unawareness of personal identity; (3) pathological preoccupation with particular inaminate objects without regard to their accepted functions; (4) sustained resistance to change in the environment; (5) abnormal perceptual experience; (6) excessive anxiety; (7) speech that did not develop, was lost, or is not used in meaningful communication; (8) distortion in motility patterns; and (9) a background of apparent intellectual retardation in which there are islets of normal or exceptional intellectual function or skill.

Rimland (1964), following Kanner, postulated autism as a "unique psychosis" distinct from childhood schizophrenia and mental retardation. He developed extensive criteria, operationalized in the form of a checklist, by which to make this differential diagnosis. Like Kanner, he identified the child's aloneness and need for sameness as the primary features differentiating autism from other psychotic childhood illnesses. Rimland's sample also finds that autistic children have well-formed bodies, normal EEG's, normal motor coordination, and parents with high intelligence. Goldfarb (1970), in turn, has questioned the validity of these observations as having been confirmed neither by controlled studies nor by sufficiently extensive observation.

Eisenberg (1966) classified children by etiology. Of two major categories in this system, the first is constituted of disorders associated with demonstrable brain-tissue pathology. They are the toxic psychoses, metabolic psychoses, degenerative psychoses (e.g., Schilder's Disease, Heller's Disease), infectious psychoses, dysrhythmic psychoses, traumatic psychoses (e.g., cerebral injury), the neoplastic psychoses. The second category, the functional psychoses, consists of those cases in which evidence of tissue pathology is not manifest, but Eisenberg emphasizes that organic bases cannot be ruled out. There are five diagnoses: autism, with onset in the first year; childhood schizophrenia, with onset after about eight years; folie à deux; manic-depressive psychosis, not observed until twelve years; and early childhood psychosis, a general term which includes Bender's childhood schizophrenia, Rank's (1955) atypical child syndrome, and Eisenberg's nonspecific category of psychosis associated with maturation failure.

## A Second Generation of Modern Investigation

Fish and Ritvo (1979) mark 1956 as beginning a second generation of twentieth-century investigations into childhood psychosis in which the emphasis has been primarily on the potential organic substrate of the illness. These studies can be divided by their focus into neurological, biochemical, genetic, complications of gestation and delivery, and neurointegrative developmental investigations. Underlying much of this research is an attempt to validate scientifically the organic speculations of an earlier generation of modern scientists. For example, Goldfarb (1956) studied an "organic" subgroup of childhood psychosis sufferers selected on the basis of IQ impairment, "soft" or nonspecific neurologic signs, and other overt physical defects. This group had more adequate families than a nonorganic group of patients, a finding which led Goldfarb to postulate a complementary series of constitutional and environmental factors which would lead to a schizophrenic outcome.

Fish (1959, 1961, 1963) has been engaged in a longitudinal study of the developmental differences between children born to schizophrenic and nonpsychotic mothers. She combined neurological and intelligence test data to study what she referred to as "integrative disorders of development." In the footsteps of Bender, she felt that these were vulnerable or genetically predisposed infants with a global neurointegrative defect; for these infants, claims Fish, the ultimate prognosis depends on the severity of the intrinsic defect and the nature of the child's experiences.

Ornitz and Ritvo (1976) have published a series of studies of biochemical and neurological deviations in autistic children which they feel lie at the root of the illness and which may also establish a link between autism and childhood schizophrenia. In addition to the criteria of noncommunicative speech and bizarre and stereotyped behaviors, Ornitz and Ritvo require for the diagnosis of autism evidence of unmodulated visual, vestibular, and auditory perceptual response, and irregular maturation in these areas. They thus make more sophisticated Kanner's and Bender's criteria.

Neurologically focused studies of psychotic children in the late 1960s and 1970s (Werry, 1972; Sameroff & Chandler, 1975; Knobloch & Pasamanick, 1975) have attempted to relate a lesion in the brain or a structural deficit in the central nervous system with subsequent psychopathology. Such an occurrence—as yet not discovered—may directly produce a behavior disorder, a minor neurologic deficit, a latent predisposition or vulnerability to a subsequent catalyst, or a fulminating developmental failure in the form of an early-onset childhood psychosis.

Genetic research has also accelerated, initially under the influence of work on the hereditary basis of adult schizophrenia (Kety, 1968). Nonetheless, concrete findings have been limited. Still, two important strands of genetic research are relevant to etiological theories of childhood psychopathology. The first, based on studies of individual differences in temperament in infants (Thomas et al., 1968), posits genetic bases for these behavioral differences. The second, based on studies of the transmission of schizophrenia (Kety, 1968), investigates the potential increased likelihood adults and children with schizophrenic relatives have for developing schizophrenia themselves. In addition to current unclarity about the existence of increased genetically determined rates of illness, there are other unanswered questions. What is the prior generation's expression of symptoms? Which relatives would carry the genetic marker? How does the transmission and expression process take place? And are there different chromosomal markers for different types of childhood psychosis if there is, in fact, genetic transmission?

The study of twins is a strategy, based on innate genetic similarities in siblings, that has been used to distinguish the developmental effects of constitution and rearing in infants. Studying a series of normal twinships, the work of Thomas et al. (1968) and Chess et al. (1968) indicated that temperament had an hereditary component: monozygotic pairs of twins were more alike than dizygotic pairs, and the dizygotic pairs were, as predicted, no more alike than nontwin siblings. Further, no large differences were found within monozygotic twins. The strongest evidence for a genetic component was for the temperamental characteristics of degree of infant activity, approach-withdrawal, and adaptability. Evidence that temperamental intensity, stimulus threshold, and mood have a genetic basis appeared in only the first three years of life; and evidence for genetic influence was stronger in the first year of life for all of the temperamental characteristics than in subsequent years.

Temperament, as used by Chess and Thomas, describes innate characteristics which influence the child's behavior. Thus a baby can be described as active, avoidant, intense, for example. These are behavioral referents of underlying psychobiological processes. Thus, if certain temperamental characteristics are genetically based, especially in the first year of life, they would determine to a degree the type of infant with whom the mother is interacting. This leads to the concept of mother-infant "fit"; for example, an intense, easily disorganized infant and a mother with low tolerance for this behavior would be a poor "fit" that could contribute to a distressing relationship. By contrast, a baby with a predisposition toward unadaptability, intensity, and a low threshold for excitability may be cared for in such a way that these constitutional characteristics do not lead to individual or dyadic behavioral parent-child disorganization. Chess and Thomas theorize that although these temperamental characteristics have a strong genetic component, they are not immutable. The maternal caretaking environment may considerably modify these qualities (Rutter, 1977).

With particular reference to schizophrenia, genetic studies (Kety, 1968) suggest that there may be a genotype that will manifest itself in the adult illness under any circumstances; and a different genotype that requires particular environmental or maturational stresses for the expression of the schizophrenic illness. However, evidence for the genetic transmission of the childhood psychoses is more rudimentary. An overview by Fish and Ritvo (1978) reports that schizophrenic children and "preschizophrenic" children suffering an early childhood psychosis have families with an increased number of schizophrenic relatives. By contrast, Rutter reports (1970) that the rate of autistic children with psychotic relatives is similar to that of the general population.

Physical trauma to the developing fetus or neonate has also received attention in recent years. Torrey et al. (1966), Bender et al. (1972), and Fish (1968) have recognized that complications of pregnancy are significantly more frequent in children who develop an early-onset childhood psychosis than in normal children. Further, pregnancy complications are more frequent in the histories of autistic children than in children developing symbiotic psychosis of childhood. According to Fish and Ritvo (1979), pregnancy complications appear to add a nonspecific impairment, which includes a lowering of IQ, to the overall clinical picture. This may be similar to an apparent, nonspecific influence of gestational problems seen in many other types of disturbed children.

## Conclusion

Genetics and neonatology bring us to date in this historical overview of the development of the field of childhood psychosis. The sixteenth century saw the beginning of attempts to understand the puzzle of the illness, and each historical period exploited the scientific paradigms and tools of its time. While some theories have been discarded—and others will certainly be in the future—knowledge has grown with respect to etiology, nosology, and treatment. Although biologically directed technology is the most recent advance, psychologically based research that draws from psychoanalysis, psychiatry, and developmental psychology continues its major role in the investigation of the childhood psychoses. Our own research, which this volume describes, is in this latter tradition. Its discussion may fill in another piece of the puzzle that is psychosis.

# Chapter 2

# The Diagnosis of Childhood Psychosis

The nosology of the severe psychopathology of childhood is complex. In traversing the historical developments of the subfield of child psychiatry that investigates childhood psychosis, we saw in Chapter 1 how diagnostic categories were often shaped by theoretical orientation as well as by the knowledge available at the time. Chapter 1 also outlined a history of gradual refinement in the description and comprehension of childhood psychosis. This chapter follows from the last, but its purpose is to delineate and organize more thoroughly the different disorders which comprise the syndromes of childhood psychosis into a highly useful nomenclature for both clinician and researcher alike.

The lexicon of diagnostic categories we outline builds on the work of previous child psychiatrists and shares many similarities to the recent *Diagnostic and Statistical Manual III (DSM-III)* (American Psychiatric Association, 1980), but it also incorporates key findings of the Early Natural History of Childhood Psychosis Project. Thus we feel that the nosology presented here makes useful and increasingly discrete distinctions between syndromes while remaining relatively simple and easy to use. This is the nomenclature we shall use consistently for the remainder of the book.

The term *childhood psychosis* itself is a superordinate concept which encompasses a range of the most severe disorders of total personality functioning during the years prior to adolescence. Psychosis is specifically a profound behavioral impairment: a disintegration of or arrest in development of the personality, failure of reality testing, and social isolation. And childhood psychosis is the general organizing umbrella for several syndromes which are differentiated by behavior or symptomatology, age of onset, diverse clinical course, a distinction between organic and functional etiology ("functional" indicating cases where there is no concrete evidence of organic central-nervous-system dysfunction), and sometimes by an understanding of intrapsychic developmental differences in different syndromes.

Pulling these strands together, Creak and the British Working Party on classification (1961, 1963) listed the essential findings in children suffering a childhood psychosis:

### TABLE 2-1    *Diagnosis of childhood psychosis (Creak, 1961)*

**1.** Gross and sustained *impairment of emotional relationships* with people. This includes the more usual aloofness and the empty clinging (so-called symbiosis): also abnormal behavior towards other people as persons, such as using them impersonally. Difficulty in mixing and playing with other children is often outstanding and long-lasting.

**2.** *Apparent unawareness of the child's own personal identity* to a degree inappropriate to age. This may be seen in abnormal behavior towards the self, such as posturing or exploration and scrutiny of parts of the body. Repeated self-directed aggression, sometimes resulting in actual damage, may be another aspect of this lack of integration (see also point 5), as is also the confusion of personal pronouns (see point 7).

**3.** *Pathological preoccupation with particular objects* or certain characteristics of them, without regard to their accepted functions.

**4.** *Sustained resistance to change in the environment* and a striving to maintain or restore sameness. In some instances behavior appears to aim at producing a state of perceptual monotony.

**5.** *Abnormal perceptual experience* (in the absence of discernible organic abnormality) is implied by excessive, diminished, or unpredictable response to sensory stimuli—for example, visual and auditory avoidance (see also points 2 and 4), insensitivity to pain and temperature.

**TABLE 2-1**  *Diagnosis of childhood psychosis (Creak, 1961)* (continued)

**6.** Acute, excessive, and seemingly illogical *anxiety* is a frequent phenomenon. This tends to be precipitated by change, whether in material environment or in routine, as well as by temporary interruption of a symbiotic attachment to persons or things (compare to points 3 & 4, and also 1 & 2).

**7.** *Speech* may have been lost or never acquired, or may have failed to develop beyond a level appropriate to an earlier stage. There may be confusion of personal pronouns (see point 2), echolalia, or other mannerisms of use and diction. Though words or phrases may be uttered, they may convey no sense of ordinary communication.

**8.** *Distortion in motility patterns*—for example, (a) excess as in hyperkinesis, (b) immobility as in catatonia, (c) bizarre postures, or ritualistic mannerisms, such as rocking and spinning (themselves or objects).

**9.** *A background of serious retardation in which islets of normal,* near normal, or exceptional *intellectual function or skill may appear.*

The British Working Party definition, however, treats childhood psychosis in its general sense as an umbrella term, utilizing descriptive behavioral criteria to sort children into the diagnostic category. Shortly afterward, Eisenberg (1966) provided a classification which broke the childhood psychoses down into organic illnesses and functional illnesses; and the functional psychoses were further subdivided into autism, childhood schizophrenia, folie à deux, manic-depressive illness, and an undifferentiated category which he called "early childhood psychosis." This classification emphasizes etiology and age of onset, while the earlier British Working Party symptom descriptions continue to be useful in their delineation of the behaviors of many of these children. The Eisenberg scheme is as follows:

**TABLE 2-2**  *Classification of Childhood Psychosis (Eisenberg, 1966)*

**1.** The toxic psychoses
**2.** Metabolic psychoses
**3.** Degenerative psychoses (e.g., Schilder's, Heller's diseases)
**4.** Infectious psychoses
**5.** Dysrhythmic psychoses

**TABLE 2-2** *Classification of Childhood Psychosis*
*(Eisenberg, 1966)* **(continued)**

6. Traumatic psychoses (e.g., cerebral injury)
7. Neoplastic psychoses
8. Functional psychoses:
   a. Autism—onset in the first year of life
   b. Childhood schizophrenia—onset after about 8 years; satisfies the diagnostic criteria for schizophrenia in the adult
   c. Folie à deux—in which a presumably healthy child reflects the symptoms of a psychotic person with whom he has a close relationship
   d. Rare manic-depressive psychosis—not observed before 12 years
   e. Early childhood psychosis—an undifferentiated category to include such nonspecific categories as the atypical child syndrome (Rank, 1955), psychoses associated with maturation failure (Eisenberg, 1966), childhood psychosis (Boatman & Szurek, 1960), childhood schizophrenia (Bender, 1947), psychosis on top of mental defect (Kraepelin, 1919)

Most recently *DSM-III* has taken a fresh look at diagnosis. The general term—formerly childhood psychosis—becomes *Pervasive Developmental Disorder*. When the illness arises between thirty months and twelve years of age, it is *Childhood Onset Pervasive Developmental Disorder;* before thirty months of age, the diagnosis is *Autism*. *DSM-III* allows for partial and atypical manifestations of these syndromes, but it does not include a diagnosis of Childhood Schizophrenia within the section on Disorders First Evident in Childhood. It does however indicate that children may show the same features of illness as adult schizophrenics—delusions, hallucinations, incoherence, or marked loosening of associations—and the same features as adults suffering affective disorders. *DSM-III* emphasizes groupings of abnormal behaviors and age of onset without consideration of etiology in its nomenclature for childhood psychosis, as follows:

**TABLE 2-3** *Infantile Autism, full syndrome (DSM-III)*

Differential diagnosis. Hearing Impairment; Mental Retardation; Childhood Onset Pervasive Developmental Disorder; Developmental Language Disorder, Receptive Type; Schizophrenia.
DIAGNOSTIC CRITERIA
A. Onset before 30 months
B. Pervasive lack of responsiveness to other people (autism)

*28*

**TABLE 2-3** *Infantile Autism, full syndrome (DSM-III)* **(continued)**

C. Gross deficits in language development
D. If speech is present, peculiar speech patterns such as immediate and delayed echolalia, metaphorical language, pronominal reversal
E. Bizarre responses to various aspects of the environment, e.g., resistance to change, peculiar interest in or attachments to animate or inanimate objects
F. Absence of delusions, hallucinations, loosening of associations, and incoherence as in Schizophrenia

---

**TABLE 2-4** *Childhood Onset Pervasive Developmental Disorder, full syndrome present (DSM-III)*

---

DIAGNOSTIC CRITERIA

A. Gross and sustained impairment in social relationships, e.g., lack of appropriate affective responsivity, inappropriate clinging, asociality, lack of empathy
B. At least three of the following:
    1. sudden excessive anxiety manifested by such symptoms as free-floating anxiety, catastrophic reactions to everyday occurrences, inability to be consoled when upset, unexplained panic attacks
    2. constricted or inappropriate affect, including lack of appropriate fear reactions, unexplained rage reactions, and extreme mood lability
    3. resistance to change in the environment (e.g., upset if dinner time is changed), or insistence in doing things in the same manner every time (e.g., putting on clothes always in the same order)
    4. oddities of motor movement, such as peculiar posturing, peculiar hand or finger movements, or walking on tiptoe
    5. abnormalities of speech, such as questionlike melody, monotonous voice
    6. hyper- or hypo-sensitivity to sensory stimuli, e.g., hyperacusis
    7. self-mutilation, e.g., biting or hitting self, head banging
C. Onset of the full syndrome after 30 months of age and before 12 years of age
D. Absence of delusions, hallucinations, incoherence, or marked loosening of associations

---

**TABLE 2.5** *Atypical Pervasive Developmental Disorder (DSM-III)*

---

This category should be used for children with distortions in the development of multiple basic psychological functions that are involved in the development of social skills and language and that cannot be classified as either Infantile Autism or Childhood Onset Pervasive Developmental Disorder.

---

Every nosologic approach offers some clarity, but each system also obfuscates important distinctions. Thus *DMS-III*—while useful from the point of view of consistency in focusing just on empirical observations of behavior and in calling attention to the developmental level of impaired behavior—omits consideration of some important data which is currently available. For example, it does not include the relatively recent recognition of symbiotic psychopathology (Mahler, 1968); or our own descriptions of failures of maturation of affective facial expression and impaired progression through the sensorimotor stages of cognitive development in the first two years of life. Therefore our own approach to the nomenclature of functional psychosis (which inevitably also loses clarity in some areas relative to other classifications) first subdivides childhood psychosis into *early childhood psychosis* for those illnesses appearing before six years of age, and *later childhood psychosis* for those appearing after age 6—childhood schizophrenia, manic-depressive disease, and folie à deux. We further subdivide early childhood psychosis into three major syndromes— Autism, Symbiotic Psychosis of Childhood, and Mixed Form of Early Childhood Psychosis. Autism has the same features as in *DSM-III* (and is very close to the syndrome originally described by Kanner), but Pervasive Developmental Disorder of Early Childhood, we feel, can be more informatively treated with the two diagnoses above (Symbiotic Psychosis of Childhood and Mixed Form). A further reason for preferring Mixed Form of Early Childhood Psychosis to Pervasive Developmental Disorder is that, in our research and clinical experience (see especially Chapters 6 and 9), illness often begins in the second year of life while Pervasive Developmental Disorder is said to be fully present only after thirty months. In addition, the developmental emphasis of the term obscures the fact that it shares with other psychotic syndromes the profound disconnection with reality. The Reactive Attachment Disorder of Infancy (*DSM-III*) must be distinguished from the early childhood psychoses (just as from Pervasive Developmental Disorders in *DSM-III*). It has also been known as Deprivation Syndrome of Childhood, and it may show features of profound developmental arrest similar to autism from which it must also be distinguished. Reactive Attachment Disorder of Infancy occurs in the first twelve months in children who have been severely neglected. They are thus unable to form affectional bonds to others for reasons of deprivation rather than organic deficit; and they may not visually track faces, smile, show reciprocity, anticipatory alerting, or reaching. Their cry may be weak, and there may be hypomotility, flaccidity, excessive sleep, poor rooting and grasping, and failure to gain weight. This syndrome is not a psychosis because signs of reality break or self- or other distortion are absent. Rather, it is a profound developmental failure. Unlike autism, when these babies do receive nurturing, their development makes rapid strides.

When one surveys our own as well as others' schemes for classifying childhood psychoses, it is useful to notice the various psychiatric traditions that contribute to nosology and their diagnostic implications. Each tradition operates with somewhat different assumptions about the mechanisms which underlie these profound emotional illnesses of childhood. Thus there are (1) etiologically based diagnoses; (2) structurally based classifications, which emphasize the intactness or deficiency of psychological structures such as the ego; (3) psychodynamically oriented terms; (4) descriptive diagnoses; and (5) developmental diagnoses.

Eisenberg's scheme illustrates most directly the etiological approach by separating the childhood psychoses into those that are organically based and those that are functional because there is no known brain damage which can be validated by physical examination or laboratory tests. This does not rule out organic factors on two fronts: first, constitutional factors may make a child more vulnerable to environmental trauma, as we suggest, especially in Chapters 9 and 10; second, the absence of signs of localizing neurologic disturbance does not rule out its as-yet-to-be-demonstrated existence in children classified as functionally disturbed. Workers such as Bender (1959), Fish (1968), and Ritvo and Ornitz (1976) have been staunch and persuasive advocates of this point of view.

The descriptive approach grows from Kraeplinian classificatory psychiatry. Aberrant behaviors receive careful description and grouping into clusters which define specific syndromes. This characterizes Kanner's original description of autism, the work of Creak and his associates, and it is the cornerstone upon which *DSM-III* is built. In addition to grouping behaviors, *DSM-III* also includes a recognition of how groups of symptoms are connected with similar disease histories and responses to treatment. However, there seems to be an implicit assumption in descriptive diagnosis that we do not understand underlying causes and mechanisms of illnesses. Behaviors are referents for something deeper, but what?

In many ways the structural diagnostic approach addresses this. It grows from psychoanalytic metapsychological theory, and looks at internal psychological structures and their role in the cause of illness.

It is closely aligned with psychodynamic diagnosis which, in turn, derives from psychoanalytic clinical theory which studies the interplay between the psychological apparatus and the environment. Both combine to seek the *meaning* to the child at both the unconscious and conscious levels (one of the first tenets of psychoanalytic metapsychology was that the mind was structured into a conscious and unconscious level) of the disturbed behaviors which are but an external display. In this scheme, diagnosis derives from an understanding in a given child of the state of his ego boundaries, his animate and inanimate object relations, the nature of his parental introjects and identifications, the state of his ego and drive development, and the defenses available to mediate against drives and their associated affects. For the child, there is a *significance* to his symptoms that can be translated into feelings about his caretakers and the psychological structures and mechanisms that mediate the emotional interactions.

Examples of structural diagnostic terms are "regression of ego functions" in Symbiotic Psychosis of Childhood and "severe distortions in ego or identity development and confusion of boundaries" in Mixed Form of Early Childhood Psychosis. Psychodynamically derived formulations are "regression on separation from the mother" and "impaired relationships" in Symbiotic Psychosis of Childhood; guilt and self-esteem problems in manic-depressive illness; and a child's identification with a psychotic person in folie à deux. Such phenomena as anxiety, aggression, and clinging clearly have both descriptive and psychodynamic implications. This multiplicity of potential interpretations is consistent with clinical psychoanalytic tradition. When a psychodynamically oriented worker looks at a symptom, he believes it to be multidetermined—that is, the same behavior can represent a multitude of meanings for different patients.

The last-mentioned diagnostic tradition is the classification of children developmentally. Symbiotic Psychosis of Childhood is equally a structural/psychodynamic diagnosis and a developmental diagnosis, for it highlights a baby's failure to emerge from the symbiotic tie with the mother toward the end of the first year and to pursue the separation-individuation stage of psychological growth in the second and third years of life. *DSM-III* also emphasizes development, although essentially descriptively, by attempting to change our perception of the major disorders of childhood away from seeing them as psychotic illnesses and toward the direction of maturational illness (Pervasive Developmental Disorders). In spite of this *DSM-III* inclination, psychosis remains psychosis. But the developmental classification bent may have fortuitously drawn us closer to recognizing the etiologic significance of failures and traumas at psychological developmental stages that lead to maturational arrests, psychotic defenses, and restitutive phenomena such as hallucinations (which restore a false world to a traumatized child). Such findings are at the core of our own research which follows in succeeding chapters.

Finally, the diagnosis Mixed Form of Early Childhood Psychosis shares all of the diagnostic traditions, but highlights developmental concepts in that children suffering Mixed Form of Early Childhood Psychosis frequently cannot be given a more specific diagnosis precisely because *their development is very uneven.* In several areas they may show age-appropriate ego functions, and in others, developmental arrests, regressions, or other major symptoms. Rank (1955) described this well for her category of atypical child syndrome, which our Mixed Form incorporates. Likewise *DSM-III* seems to acknowledge this possibility with the subcategory Atypical Pervasive Developmental Disorder.

Even though the psychoanalytically informed nosologies clarify the meaning and psychological mechanisms for symptoms, and developmental terms point to stage disruptions, the basic causes of the psychoses remain hazy, as they also are for those workers seeking biochemical/neurologic factors. The organicist turns to the laboratory to obtain information about etiology, and the psychoanalytic/dynamically oriented worker employs therapeutic skills with psychotic children and their families in order to classify and unravel what the symptoms are communicating. And at the same time that the clinician is engaging in the therapeutic endeavor, he or she frequently begins to understand critical factors in the etiology of a particular child's illness. In fact, a hallmark of this kind of diagnosis is that a clinician at the least must spend long hours of evaluation with a child to make a diagnosis, and at best, makes assessments such as, for example, Symbiotic Psychosis of Childhood or "disturbance of drive development and defense," through understanding the process of a child's play and his or her transference distortions in the treatment. Cases 4, 9, and 10 in Chapter 6 illustrate how the therapeutic process with family and child can produce precise descriptions of intrapsychic distortions. A case report by Bonnard (1967) describes this still more subtly.

Because psychoanalytic diagnoses require an unusually precise ordering of all the data available—phenomenologic observation, developmental history, and understanding of the therapeutic process— and because they are based on a theory of the unconscious and the unfolding of hypothesized developmental phases, it is sometimes difficult to achieve reliability among different workers. By contrast, descriptively oriented diagnoses such as *DSM-III* are more easily validated and reliable since they posit a necessary and sufficient cluster of symptoms for making a diagnosis. In fact, it is instructive to think of structural/dynamic/developmental labels as being the diagnosis of an individual child, and of descriptive diagnosis as the label of an illness. When viewed this way, the different kinds of diagnostic processes are not mutually exclusive.

Our own classification, which Tables 2-6, 2-7, 2-8, and 2-9 outline, is an amalgam of the several traditions, a combination we feel is valuable because these traditions are mutually informative and supportive. The nomenclature as we use it balances clinical functionality, continuity with the history of diagnosis in child psychiatry, and incorporation of previously unavailable information.

We have applied our nosology the following way in The Early Natural History of Childhood Psychosis Study. In Chapter 6, where ten case histories appear in detail, with the child's name at the beginning of the case report, we provide our own diagnosis in the framework of our nomenclature. The label that a child's therapist or institution originally applied to the child appears in the history section of the case. There is no certainty that this historical diagnosis was always accurate, and some of the children received different diagnoses at different times because of the views of different clinicians about the changing picture of the symptomatology. In our nomenclature for early childhood psychosis (before age 6), there is autism, symbiotic psychoses of childhood, and mixed form of early childhood psychosis. The diagnosis we give the child comes from all of the data available to us—the observation of the longitudinal film data, histories and

**Table 2-6** *Classification of Early Childhood Psychosis (Massie-Rosenthal)*

| Early (before 6 years) | Later (after 6 years) |
|---|---|
| Autism / Mixed Form of Early Childhood Psychosis | Childhood Schizophrenia / Folie à deux |
| Symbiotic Psychosis of Childhood | Manic-Depressive Illness |

**Table 2-7  Early Childhood Psychosis: Autism**

| | |
|---|---|
| From *DSM-III* | • Onset before 30 months<br>• Pervasive lack of responsiveness to other people<br>• Gross deficits in language development<br>• If speech present, peculiar speech patterns such as immediate and delayed echolalia, metaphorical language, pronominal reversals<br>• Bizarre responses to various aspects of the environment, e.g., resistance to change, peculiar interest in or attachments to inanimate or animate objects<br>• Absence of delusions, hallucinations, loosening of associations, and incoherence as in schizophrenia |
| From Creak (1961) | • Islets of normal or near normal intellectual function or skill<br>• Distortion in motility such as excessive movement, immobility, posturing or ritualistic mannerisms (rocking, spinning, hand and finger movements) |
| From Massie-Rosenthal | • Failure of facial (and verbal) expression to mature in 2nd year toward communication of mood, affect, intention and meaning; instead immature lability persists<br>• Progression through the Sensorimotor stages of cognitive development slowed or arrested in first 2 years |

**Table 2-8  Early Childhood Psychosis: Symbiotic Psychosis of Childhood**

| | |
|---|---|
| From Massie-Rosenthal | • Mood marked more by irritability and depression than by withdrawal, from infancy |
| Largely from Mahler (1968) | • Onset in 2nd to 4th year<br>• Panic, tantrums and desperate clinging at separation from mother<br>• Severe regression of ego functions when mother absent<br>• Bizarre and obsessive preoccupation<br>• Severely impaired relationships with other children and adults; aloof and/or anxious<br>• Extreme vulnerability to frustration as toddler |

**Table 2-9** *Early Childhood Psychosis: Mixed Form of Early Childhood Psychosis*

| | |
|---|---|
| From *DSM-III* (Pervasive Developmental Disorder) | • Onset after 1 year<br>• A syndrome which may have some features of autism and symbiotic psychosis of childhood, but is not sufficiently characteristic of either; nor is it simply a partial or residual expression of autism or symbiotic psychosis<br>• Severe impairment in social relations, e.g., inappropriate affect, clinging, asociality, lack of empathy, extensive fears and rages<br>• Sudden excessive anxiety and upset<br>• Resistance to change in environment<br>• Oddities in motor movement<br>• Speech abnormalities, such as hyperquestioning and melodious or monotonous voice<br>• Self-mutilation or head-banging |
| Largely from Creak (1961) | • Severe distortions in ego or identity development characterized by confusion of boundaries of the self and others, marked by dangerous aggression to the self or others, and by speech reversals<br>• Islets of normal intellectual function and social skill |
| From Massie/Rosenthal | • Progression through the Sensorimotor stages of cognitive development slowed or arrested in the first 2 years |

medical records of the children and project questionnaires, accounts of the therapeutic process, firsthand therapy in some cases, and firsthand interviews with families and patients in some cases. In sections of the project where we do more standardized empirical studies (Chapter 7 and 8), in order to work statistically with small numbers of cases we group all the children into either autism or early childhood psychosis. This is a more standardized descriptive categorization based simply on behaviors. Thus a psychodynamic/structural diagnosis is converted into the descriptive category which most nearly approximates it. For example, symbiotic psychoses of childhood often become early childhood psychosis.

À propos of diagnosis and syndromes, another interesting observation emerged from the case studies in The Childhood Psychosis Project. A few of the children who clearly suffered one of the early childhood psychoses prior to age six, after six years developed hallucinations and delusions, cardinal symptoms of schizophrenia. The finding that these children were both victims of early childhood psychosis *and* childhood schizophrenia raises questions about possible connections between the syndromes and the longitudinal course of the illnesses from earliest life to later childhood. The case reports, together with the discussion chapters, shed some light on these queries.

*Chapter 3*

# Normal Development—The Earliest Mother-Child Interaction

Chapters 3 and 4 outline the normative development of the infant. Chapter 3 treats the somatic, perceptual, cognitive, auditory, and social capacities, and Chapter 4 focuses on the formation of psychological, that is to say, intrapsychic structures. Such a normative baseline is important for (1) understanding the incongruities that the childhood psychosis cases present which distinguish them from the normal, (2) considering aberrancies in intrapsychic development which we hypothesize to have occurred in the childhood psychosis children, although they were not directly observable, and (3) providing a starting point for the building of etiological hypotheses of childhood psychoses in Chapters 9 and 10 regarding the nature of psychic trauma, the timing, and the outcome.

In particular we review here studies of the past two decades that address infant development in the important parameters of state of arousal, reflex activity, tactility, hearing, vision, sleep, cognition, affect, and social interaction. The understanding of key elements in the early development of physiologic and psychological apparatus shows the infant to be an active, stimulus-seeking being who is ready to interact with its animate and inanimate environment in complex ways. In addition, it points to critical periods and processes wherein disturbance may be especially disorganizing for subsequent growth. In addition, an appreciation emerges of the subtle, yet profound interface between the infant's own regulatory capacities and the external (mother and environment) regulators which influence infant behavior and growth.

Our sources for this review come from the fields of embryology, neurology, neurophysiology, neuroanatomy, ethology, developmental psychology, and psychiatry. Until the past few decades, the infant was seen as a passive, undifferentiated creature who functioned at a purely biological level. Communication to the mother was for the purpose of indicating need states. However, within the past two decades evidence points to the newborn and the infant (the first two weeks and the first year of life, respectively) as organized and purposive in behavior and able to communicate both need and affect states. The first school of infancy researchers in the late 1950s and 1960s were primarily interested in the caretaker's shaping role since the interaction was thought to be unidirectional—from mother to infant (R. Q. Bell, 1968). With increased information on the capacities of the infant, the influence of the infant on the caretaker became the focus of study (Lewis & Rosenblum, 1974). This was the second school of infancy research. The third focused on the mother and infant as an interactional system (Sander, 1975), each having separate competencies which affect the other's behavior. Thus the infant's capacity to communicate to the mother as well as the mother's ability to "understand" her baby's behavior and respond empathically point toward their relationship as an important impetus for the infant's development.

## Transitions in Development

In considering the parameters of infant behavior, it is important to take into account the significance of maturational and developmental shifts. One such important shift occurs between two and three months and has important ramifications for the adaptive capacities of the infant with his environment: the transition from endogenous to exogenous control of behavior. Some definitions are in order. "Endogenous" refers to behavior which is internally activated and maintained. Neurologically, this is generally behavior under midbrain, autonomic and peripheral nervous system control. While endogenous behavior is not dependent upon external stimuli for activation and maintenance, that does not imply that the infant is shut off from external stimuli: the infant still interacts with the environment; however, the force of its biobehavioral system is internally based. The explanation for the predominance of endogenous control in the first two to three months is based on its function in facilitating neurological growth. During this period, the central system is under limbic system or brain stem control. Endogenous stimulation, which is kept relatively constant through the processes of the basic sleep-rest activity cycle (Sterman, 1972), facilitates a maximal rate of cortical neuronal firing. At about two to three months, a major internal organizational shift occurs from brainstem to forebrain control of the central nervous system. At this point the infant has the capacity for more complex behaviors related to external stimulation. While the specific changes in each behavior system are traced below, it is important to note the existence and timing of this transitional phase, for it has many implications for the infant's behavior. To summarize the nature of the change in a simple way: it represents the infant's completion of an important phase in neurological maturation, an achievement in internal biobehavioral organization which allows the baby the capacity to turn more to the outside world. This internal structure-building leads to external function.

Concomitant changes in sleep patterns, positive affect, a decline in fussiness, and increased responsivity by the baby to its surroundings mark the major changes of this transitional period of life. This time, a nodal point in which there are observable behavioral referents of underlying neuromaturational processes, has important implications for developmental psychopathology. First, infants with congenital neurologic problems may manifest the symptomatology of illness initially at this point with a failure to mature neurologically. Until this transitional phase, prodromal signs may appear in the form of hyper- or hypotonicity and irritability. When such signs continue, they may provide subtle, then more overt manifestations of the beginning of psychopathology with a neurological or organic etiology.

Second, the infant who handles the transition from endogenous to exogenous control in good fashion develops the capacity for self-regulation and becomes a more active responsive participant in the mother-infant interaction. Such an infant will be better able to modulate impending internal disorganization because of its increasingly structured neurological system. The baby at this point can be an increasingly rich source of pleasure to the parents. From the interactional perspective, such an infant will be easier for an inexperienced and/or anxious mother to handle. Alternatively, less anxious and sensitive mothers may facilitate optimal behavior from the infant by their interventions; the infant whose behavior is exogenously controlled, that is, the baby who has made the major shift from midbrain to more cortical control of behavior, will be more available to the mother, more attuned to her cues for interaction. Thus, the sensitive mother and organized infant would interact in a highly synchronous way (Chappell, Sander, & Rosenthal, 1976).

Third, the infant who is slow to make the transition in control of biological rhythms has an effect on the mother. An anxious mother may be concerned about her baby's development and this, in turn, is reflected in caretaking behavior. The anxiety is communicated to the infant through the various interactional modalities of touch, vision, hearing, and holding. In particular, mothers may become concerned about sleep patterns when a baby does not "settle" into a regular pattern of day wakefulness and night-time sleep. If the sleep-wakefulness behavioral system remains in premature rhythms, it is both clearly manifest to the parent and a distressing disruption of their own routine. It can extend the early postnatal adaptation, which normally stabilizes by six weeks. The infant who is "slow" in making the transition from endogenous to exogenous control may very well be within the range of normal neuromaturation, and later accelerate developmentally; however, the baby's slowness may effect the parental response in a way that has important consequences for the development of later psychopathology in the child (Sperling, 1982). Parental tension is normal, but extreme anxiety, impatience, or anger may translate into untoward caretaking and affective interaction with the infant. This may surface in a lack of sensitivity to the baby's cues, producing in the infant the sense that its needs are not contingently responded to. This can lead to a growing experience on the part of the infant that its behavior has no predictable effect on the environment. According to Lewis and Goldberg (1969), lack of contingency is the root of helplessness. Although lack of contingency so early in life is not irreversible, there is the potential for an etiological point of illness to be laid down by such interaction, predicated by the parents' response to the infant's slow or disturbed maturational development. Noncontingent caretaking may elicit defensive behaviors in the infant that become part of the baby's repertoire of social interactions and that may also form the basis for subsequent severe childhood emotional illness. How specific defense behaviors unfold is described in Chapter 10, which integrates the findings of the Project into a theory of pathologic development.

### State of Arousal

In the newborn infant, "state" refers to a constellation of physiological variables and/or behaviors which seem to repeat and be relatively stable. "State of arousal" is an important concept because it helps to measure the infant's capacity for endogenous control of physiological processes in response to both internal and external stimuli. The concept derives from systems theory (von Bertalanffy, 1960), emphasizing the constantly developing organism's equilibrium with his ever-changing environment.

Investigators have produced several descriptive systems for categorizing newborn behavioral states of arousal. All systems recognize two sleep states: an active one, with irregular respirations, rapid eye movements, and varying amounts of activity; and a quiet state, with no eye movements, regular respiration, and behavioral quiescence aside from intermittent startles. All systems also recognize two states of wakefulness: one often referred to as alert inactivity, in which there is little movement and the infant's capacity for visual attention is maximal; and alert activity, in which there is physical activity which may or may not be accompanied by fussiness. The fifth state is that of crying. These five states form the basis of systems used by Brazelton (1973) and Prechtl (1974). Boismier (1973) has added a state of "transitional sleep" which indexes a state between sleep and wakefulness. It is commonly referred to as "drowsy." Fussing is considered in Boismier's system to represent a separate state between alert activity and crying.

The significance of state is that the behavior of the newborn and young infant (up until about two months) is state-dependent. According to Wolff (1965, 1966), during the alert-inactive state the newborn is maximally capable of processing information from his environment. Maternal ministrations and stimulation leading to increased visual alertness of her infant give mother and infant more time to interact socially. This is a great source of pleasure for the mother and infant. Korner and Thoman (1970) compared six common maternal soothing interventions. They found that putting the infant to the shoulder was not only the most effective in diminishing crying, but also a potent elicitor of the visually alert state. Nearly 80 percent of the infants in their sample of forty responded with visual alertness.

### Reflexive Activity

By definition, reflexes are innate automatic movements. Prechtl and Beintema (1964) and Brazelton (1973) have extensively studied this aspect of the newborn's behavioral repertoire. Reflexive behaviors show many structured and complicated actions. The rooting reflex is a good example. It comprises the baby's sequence of orienting movements toward the breast and seizing the nipple, all toward the goal of sucking and swallowing. The series forms a well-defined coherent behavioral complex. Also in this complex are pressor movements with the hands and arms and movements of the legs.

An important question is, what are the somatopsychic pathways which trigger these reflex behavior patterns? Spitz (1955) defines two types of reflex organizations in the newborn: coenesthetic and diacritic. Coenesthetic reflexes are centered around the autonomic nervous system, and are behaviors that are responses to outside stimuli through peripheral sensory modalities such as the skin surface. At the end of the first week of life, these reflexes become more aim-directed; for example, when the mother lifts the infant from the crib, it turns its head in her direction and roots. Diacritical reflexes are not simply autonomically based, but also exist at a higher level, according to Spitz, and are effected through the cortex of the brain. They manifest themselves through peripheral sense organs—the fingers, eyes, ears, and nose. By the second or third week of life, the infant is able to coordinate several reflex actions into a coherent whole.

### Tactility

Emde and Robinson (1979) state that, except for measures of tactile thresholds, there have been few measures which index tactile sensitivity. They further feel that there has been little attempt to understand the ontogenesis of this perceptual modality, which is interesting since so much importance has been placed on touching and holding in the bonding-and-attachment literature.

Most of the research on tactile thresholds has emphasized the individual differences among newborns, distinguishing babies that are likely to respond to low or high intensities of stimulation (Bell, Weller, & Waldrop, 1971). Infants who have a high level of tactile sensitivity can maintain a given state much longer and are more capable of self-regulation. Those who have low levels can be more easily perturbed, and thus need more extrinsic control from the mother. The caretaking implications are obvious here. Those infants who are most capable of regulation of state are less dependent on extrinsic control by the caretaker and therefore less vulnerable to variabilities in caretaker environment. Low-intensity infants have graded responses, while high-intensity infants tend to have an all-or-none response.

### Auditory Perception

While old lore had it that the baby could not see at birth, there has never been any doubt that it can hear. The newborn literally startles in response to loud sounds. According to Eisenberg (1969), the newborn is responsive to sound frequencies in the range of human speech. Hutt, Lenard, and Prechtl (1969) have demonstrated that young infants respond to, and even prefer, speech-like sounds. Certainly responsiveness to speech sounds, combined with the baby's tendency to visual curiosity, places the infant in a strategic position to acquire schemas important for the development of its affective and cognitive capacities. Condon and Sander (1974) studied frame-by-frame films of infants who were being addressed by adult voices. They found that between one and four days of life infants move in synchrony with the sound of the adult voice.

Studies on the auditory capacity of the newborn have been confounded by state. Experimental control of state is important because it is known that a sound may startle or soothe, arouse or quiet, depending upon the initial state of the child, and then change the baby's level of arousal. Repetitive sounds, for example, have a soothing effect. This has led to problems in research where repetition is required to assess auditory discrimination.

### Visual Perception

From the voluminous literature on infant visual perception, we can provide an overview of the research with particular attention to the infant's occulomotor development, sensitivity to colors and changes of light intensity, and visual pursuit. We also consider visual stimuli that are interesting to the baby at different developmental phases and how the gestalt of the human face is an especially important stimulus for the infant in his developing social interaction with the mother.

*Historical Overview of Research on Infant Visual Perception*   According to Haith (1980), a major shift occurred in the study of infant visual perception around 1960. "The question of the pre-1960's changed from 'What stimuli does the newborn sense?' to that of the post 1960's, 'What information does the newborn attend to or prefer?' " (p. 10). This is an important shift, for it demonstrates an appreciation of the infant as an active seeker of information rather than a collator of events.

Fantz (1958, 1961) was a pioneer in developing techniques for studying the infant's attention to a visual stimulus: the choice of stimulus and the length of time the infant spent looking at it. One of his innovative techniques was based on the logic that we can know to what stimulus a baby attends by watching its eyes—the reflection of the perceived object appears on the baby's cornea.

By contrast, Haith's (1980) work reflects a current interest in the structure of infant attentional visual behavior toward a particular stimulus rather than in the stimulus. Thus Haith's interest in the structure of behavior is more in keeping with the most contemporary views of the behavioral sophistication of the infant as active stimulus-seeker rather than a passive creature who attends to what is presented to him. Nonetheless, in operationalizing seemingly simple questions, such as what visual stimuli attract the infant and why and how he utilizes them, both the structure of the stimulus and the behavior become important variables.

*Neuromaturational Questions of Oculomotor Development*   Haith (1973) has demonstrated that the pupillary light reflex, although minimal at birth, is indeed present in both fullterm and preterm infants. Haynes, White, and Held (1965) studied visual accommodation in the newborn and estimated that the lens appeared to be relatively fixed at a median accommodative distance of 19 cm. and gradually became adaptable over the first four months of life. On the basis of testing infants with interesting attractive stimuli, and taking into consideration state of arousal, Hershenson (1964) has found that the newborn has somewhat more flexibility of accommodation.

Studies of visual orienting indicate that the newborn can attain a focused retinal image for stimuli with visual acuity of 20/150 to 20/800. In addition, although retinal maturation continues throughout childhood, at birth there is already differentiation of the photopic ability to adjust to bright light mediated by the cones, and scotopic ability to see in dim light mediated by the rods. Additional evidence points to functional activity in the neonate's visual cortex, suggesting brain registration of images.

Haith and Campos (1977) indicate that the infant can discriminate brightness intensities in the first few months of life, achieve the focuses described above, and detect angles. The baby is also sensitive to a moving stimulus and tracks movement. It still remains controversial as to whether an infant can distinguish colors. Methodological difficulties confound the results of studies of infant color perception because colors vary in hue, and it is unclear to what the infant may be responding. Until all potential confounding variables are controlled in the color perception studies, the findings are inconclusive (Cohen et al., 1979).

The basic principle underlying early occulomotor development is that the infant keeps the firing rate of neurons in the visual cortex at a maximum level—a "preprogrammed" endogenous function—which is thought to facilitate rapid neurological development. Consequently, visual acuity improves rapidly during the first year and appears to be within the range of normal adult vision by six months to one year (Fantz et al., 1962).

### Visual Stimuli

Over the first year, there are subtle, yet rapid changes in the kind of stimuli which attract infant attention. Fantz (1961, 1963) developed two important methods for studying stimulus preference and attention time. The first, discussed above, measured the registration of the image of the presented stimulus on the cornea of the infant. The second method involved the presentation of pairs of stimuli, with the differential fixation times recorded.

Important to his studies is the concept of habituation, or response decrement. From learning theory, this concept refers to the infant's decremental visual attention to a stimulus, based on familiarity. If the stimulus is presented many times, the infant can match it to a schema which it is building up and stops attending to it. If the stimulus lacks complexity appropriate to developmental phase, the infant may not attend at all, or only once. Thus infants require novelty for attention and for new learning. To pursue this one step further, Kagan (1971) states, "A schema is a cognitive representation of an external stimulus" (p. 339). He found that two kinds of stimuli elicit maximal attention from an infant: emergent schema and variations of older schema. The former concur with established schema, while the latter amend the complexity of previously established schema. Using the corneal reflection apparatus, some of the useful findings are:

1. Newborns can perceive high contrast edges and angles (Kessen, 1972).
2. Newborns will fixate to a horizontal line as readily as a vertical line, suggesting that there is equivalent complexity in the stimulus (Haith, 1976).
3. One-month-old infants who have been presented with different shapes tend to concentrate their fixations about a single edge or angle.
4. One-month-olds shown compound figures fixate to the outer-most contours; two-month-olds rapidly moved their eyes from the outer contour to one of the internal features. These compound-figure experiments demonstrate that both extensive scanning behavior and stimulus complexity preference increase with age.

Fantz and Miranda (1975) examined newborn visual preferences for patterns with curved versus straight lines, such as a bullseye versus a straight line. When the patterns formed the contour of the stimuli, newborns looked longer at the curved lines; however, when patterns were embedded in large white squares, no consistent preferences were found. The newborn fixations stopped at the outer contour of the square. Fantz and Nevis (1967) showed that older infants of two to four months preferred curved over straight lines, whether or not they are embedded in a square.

The logic of these studies is that attention involves selective orientation to a stimulus or set of stimuli, and that identification of the characteristics of the stimuli may promote information about the underlying cognitive processes of the infant. One of the crucial stimulus characteristics which heightens infant attention, as mentioned above, is *complexity*. And as babies get older they prefer increasingly complex stimuli. For example, Brennan (1966) found a positive relationship between age and preference for checkerboard complexity.

Greenberg (1971) offers a quantitative explanation for complexity preference—complex patterns contain more information, Kagan (1971) claims that it facilitates cognitive development. Karmel and Maisel (1967) believe that complexity facilitates neurological maturation underlying the visual system, and that cognitive development gains secondarily.

## The Structure of Infant Visual Perception

Cohen et al. (1979) raise the important question of what an infant may be responding to when appearing to fixate on a stimulus. For example, when Fantz (1961) finds that an infant looks at a black-and-white schematic drawing of a face longer than at a plain surface, is the infant responding to a high contrast area, a patterned surface, or a picture of a face? Such questions about visual preference Haith (1980) believes are best answered by studying the structure of infant *visual behavior.* He states that there is meaningful structure in infants' visual activity which requires careful description, analysis, and interpretation for an adequate articulation of babies' competencies. In his work Haith asks why babies scan their visual field, why they look at contours or edges, why they engage in scanning activity that involves frequent crossing of contours, and why their scan routine is more limited in some cases than others.

Haith describes a way of thinking about visual activity that assumes visual activity is ongoing. Stimuli, then, actually constrain this behavior by causing visual fixation responses. The significant evidence that Haith presents is that babies scan in the dark, as well as when stimuli are presented to them. This indicates that the actual behavior is present in any state of wakefulness. His explanation for such behavior, and the underlying structure of infant visual behavior, is that the visual system as a whole is comprised of discrete neurophysiological subsystems having the same goal of keeping the visual cortical firing rate at a high level. Two scanning routines keep the firing rate activity high: an "ambient search routine" and an "inspection scan routine." The former serves to find targets for inspection. It governs the continuous activity of the eye movement system and gains predominant control over eye movement activity when the cortical firing rate is low. The inspection scan routine is called into play when a target is detected, and it produces contour encounters and crosses. If the inspection scan routine produces a high firing rate, then the former system is supressed, since the criterion for control is maximum cortical firing. Haith writes,

> . . . experiments indicate that alot of eye movements by newborns, or, for that matter, adults, are meaningless—not under the control of visual stimuli. Newborns will often *not* look at stimuli. Adults will often look toward a wall, a blackboard, the floor, etc. during, for example, conversations . . . these fixations do make sense if one

thinks about eye movement generators as constantly active and as meant to serve at least one function of sampling the environment and, thereby, alerting the organism to significant events and changes in the visual field (p. 120).

While Haith bases his conclusions on neurophysiological evidence, he does draw ethological implications from it. This is implicit in the quotation above in which Haith suggests that the baby's constant scanning serves to teach him or her about the environment. He further states that since the newborn is only rarely in an alert state, constant scanning during these periods allows it to acquire as much information as possible. Interestingly enough, Haith's sophisticated neurophysiological measurements of infant perceptual behavior are in agreement with Wolff's (1965) earlier findings from direct infant observation. While Wolff's underlying theoretical framework is different—psychoanalytic and ethological—he too claims that the infant initiates alert behavior by necessity. He postulates a model of the earliest months of infant development, in which the infant eats, stools, and occasionally is in periods of alert inactivity. These moments are time for maximal visual attention that allows the infant to take in as much information as possible from both the inanimate and animate environments. Wolff traces the increasingly complex development of this visual behavior over the first six weeks, indicating its tie-in with the infant's percept of the mother and consequently its importance for the development of mother-child interaction.

### Perception of Facial Schema

Since the mother-infant interaction, in particular eye gaze, is such an important component of the social process and a source of stimulation for the infant's development, the perception of faces is especially relevant. Cohen et al. (1979) raises the question of "whether the development of face perception can be described by the same general principles as other aspects of form perception, or whether, as some suggest, there is something different or unique about an infant's response to the human face" (p. 416). This is based firstly on the issue of whether there is an innate preference for the human face. According to Bowlby (1958) and other ethologically oriented investigators, there is an innate tendency for human newborns to attend to human faces. This hypothesis has not been substantiated by studies that have compared newborns' visual fixations of faces versus other stimuli. Therefore, reported preferences for faces must be explained by other stimulus characteristics, such as their complexity. Thus, when infants have been shown faces versus other fairly complex stimuli, no face preference has emerged (Herschenson, 1964). Further, neither the orientation nor the arrangement of facial features influences the attention of newborns or infants younger than two months (Fantz, 1965; Hershenson, 1964).

Second, there is the question of whether infants attend to facial features or to the whole face and how this may change with development. Recent experiments analyzing infants' patterns of eye movements as they scan faces have shown that they scan faces in a similar manner to the way in which they scan any two-dimensional object. Mauer and Salapatek (1976) reported that *one-month-olds* fixated away from the real face, spending most of the time scanning the hairline and perimeter. In contrast, *two-month-olds* spent most of their time looking at the internal features of the face and were very likely to fixate on the eyes. It is not clear whether the eyes attracted the two-month-olds because they had acquired special meaning or simply because they were the most striking internal features. Nonetheless, two-month-old's interest in the mother's inner facial features correlates with Robson's (1967) observation that infants at about six weeks are intently interested in their mother's eyes, and that is when mothers report experiencing meaningful mutual gaze for the first time.

Gibson (1969) states that an important transition in the baby's percept of the face occurs at four months. Infants begin responding to the configurations of the face as a whole rather than to individual features. At this age they show spontaneous preferences, as indicated by longer fixations or greater smiling, for regular faces over faces with their features scrambled (Kagan et al., 1969). Faces in an upright position elicit the most smiling (Watson, 1966). More realistic versions of faces seem to be preferred over less realistic ones; and realistic faces are preferred over a wide range of other nonfacial stimuli (Fantz & Nevis, 1967). Thus by about four months, children's responses to facelike stimuli depend on how closely the stimulus resembles the human visage; and by five months, infants have become even more capable of abstracting the invariant features or relationships among features in the face.

In summary, infant perception of faces seems to follow the same general course as other aspects of form or pattern perception. There is little evidence of an innate preference for human faces, and infants younger than two months seem to respond only to a few isolated contrast features. By four months, infants respond to the whole configuration of features so that arrangements of features are important factors in determining their attention. From five months, infants become increasingly adept at abstracting invariant features from faces. They notice the structure that distinguishes one face from another and what remains constant over a variety of poses. They are also able to recognize the aspects of facial expressions that remain invariant over individuals.

### Conclusion

Nonetheless, *what* the newborn sees and *when* it sees it is largely guided by the mother and other caretakers, for they provide the visual display in both animate and inanimate terms. The caretaker controls the amount of light and sources of stimuli, and she can position her face in such a way as to allow the infant maximal exposure to it. Sensitive parents have the capacity to "read" their babies' states and know how to maximize periods of alertness (Chappell, Sander, & Rosenthal, 1976). Such sensitivity facilitates both neuromaturational growth of the visual system and the social responsiveness of the infant.

We have discussed the development of the visual system extensively because vision is the major perceptual modality which facilitates normal cognitive and emotional development. Adaptively, vision is the perceptual pathway by which the infant takes in aliment from the environment and from which schema of the world are built up. In addition, as we shall see, vision can also become organized to serve maladaptive cognitive and affective functions through head turning away, gaze aversion, eye closure, and shutting down through sleep. As we elaborate on in Chapters 4 and 10, these behaviors are important in the ontogeny of defensive behaviors in infancy.

# Sleep

Sleep in infancy has been a major area of investigation. The newborn spends nearly two-thirds of its existence in sleep. This does not mean, however, that the organism is quiet during this time, for sleep is an important facilitator of central nervous system growth. Several classificatory systems describe aspects of infant sleep: slow wave and activated wave sleep as measured by the electroencephalogram (EEG); rapid eye movement (REM) and nonrapid eye movement (NREM) sleep; and quiet versus active sleep according to behavior. In addition, there is also a second cycle—the basic rest-activity cycle (BRAC)—which is different from, though related to the sleep-wakefulness cycle. Utilizing the REM-NREM classificatory system, Roffward, Muzio, and Dement (1966) estimated that the newborn spends 50 percent of sleep time in REM sleep, as compared with 30 percent at the end of the first year, and 20 percent in adolescence. With respect to why the infant spends so much of its time in REM sleep, they postulated that early in development the organism seeks out stimulation needed for neuronal growth. REM sleep possibly provides this important source of endogenous stimulation. Agreeing with the hypothesis, Emde et al. (1976) found that much of infant sleep is very active and organized into behavioral systems. In fact, sleep activity is so extensive that when they measured the output of such behaviors as eye movement, startles, and sucks by means of an air-filled mattress, the activity exceeded that observed during wakefulness.

As the first year passes, there are significant changes in the temporal organization of sleep states. Between two and three months, correlating with the shift from endogenous to exogenous behavior and forebrain development, there is a transition to longer periods of wakefulness. "Settling," the term used to describe when a baby first starts to sleep through the night, often occurs at this time. Following Kleitman's work (1963), Sterman (1972) described REM which continues into wakefulness in infants. This led him to distinguish a basic rest-activity cycle from the sleep-wakefulness cycle. Thus there is quiet sleep and REM which may occur during sleep or wakefulness. He writes, "The continued and intensified manifestations of the REM state in the infant . . . represent a more fundamental recurrent process than sleep itself, a process which continues during wakefulness" (1972, p. 177). He infers that REM and the underlying physiological processes it indexes bear little resemblance to actual sleep itself. Sterman suggests that the two cycles in infancy promote the maturation of the central nervous system, but further information is needed to fill in the mechanisms of this neuromaturational process, especially with regard to the function of quiet sleep.

Chappell and Sander (1979) brought into focus the critical interface between the role of social interaction in the regulation of infant sleep and alertness and the infant's self-regulation. Videotapes of feeding interactions in the first week of life in a series of infants' lives were examined at 15-second intervals for infant states, maternal vocalization to infant, maternal manipulation of infant posture, and proximity of infant to the mother. This led to a model of the infant's active participation in the feeding situation. In the normal course of any feeding, the infant will awaken, cry, stay awake to feed, and return to sleep. Thus a baby's shift toward alertness and maintenance of alertness was optimal following the caretaker's manipulations in the period before and during the feeding. Increasingly over the first week of life, mothers and infants synchronize alert wakefulness with important events such as feeding and periods of mutual closeness which allow the baby to nurse, hear the mother's voice, and see her face.

Furthermore, analyses of the relationship between the mother's manipulation of her infant and infant state show that there is a stability of the infant state during alert episodes. Chappell and Sander report, ". . . with each successive awakening, the infant's interaction with his environment becomes increasingly stable, thus predictable. . . . If the predictable order be shared between interacting partners, a common context is provided for the more variable content of the events which take place between them, setting up the conditions under which such events also gain a meaning common to both" (p. 106).

### Cognitive Development

The major theoretical approaches of the study of infant cognition are based on the following premise: the infant "learns" through a reciprocal interaction with its animate and inanimate environment. While the underlying explanations for cognitive development in infancy vary—from Piagetian theory to the various schools of learning theory—there are major similarities in the model of the infant as an active stimulus-seeker, and in their use of the concept of feedback loops or contingency. In this section we focus primarily on the phenomenon of contingency and its relationship to the mother-infant interaction. Contingency can be measured through first-order observations, and it is readily operationalized. Further, and most important in studies of infancy, contingency originates and evolves in an interactional context.

"Contingency" is the infant's experience that his actions have an effect on the environment. "Contingently" describes the mother's responsiveness to her infant's signals in terms of providing adequate stimulation and sensitively responding to his need and affect states. In the earliest weeks of life, the mother who responds contingently to her infant is sensitive to the infant's endogenous rhythms—the rate, tempo, and range of its behaviors (Chappell & Sander, 1979). Through continued responsiveness to her infant's cues, a mother facilitates the infant's development of a "motive" for acting that is based on the perception that his actions have consequences (Lewis & Goldberg, 1969).

Watson (1979) states that contingency is a source of potency in itself: once set in motion, the infant's memory of contingency in itself evokes further action. Memory is an important mediating variable in contingency according to Watson (1967). If the infant's memory for a contingent relationship exceeds his capacity developmentally, the infant will either habituate to the experience or shut it out. Learning will not take place. There is a finely tuned synchronous process in contingency learning. If the stimulus presentation or the mother's response temporally exceeds the infant's memory, if the stimulus is too complex or discrepant, or too simple and uninteresting, the child's growing awareness of contingency will at the least be temporarily arrested. The mother is also an extremely important mediator of contingency learning through her ability to "read" her infant's communications.

Such a mother-infant partnership in the development of contingency in the infant is what Lewis and Goldberg (1969) refer to as the "generalized expectancy model."

> The proposed model is a motivational construct developed by the infant through the mother-infant interaction. The construct is a generalized expectancy that his behavior has consequences in affecting his environment. The learning of this motive is dependent upon consistent reinforcement with short latencies (that is, before the memory trace of the infant's act is gone) . . . it is also suggested that it is in the service of the motive to control, based on the infant's expectancies that he can effect change" (pp. 94–95).

Several experiments have studied the development of contingency in relation to inanimate objects. Watson (1972) utilized a paradigm in which infants could control aspects of a mobile, such as its sound and movement, via an air-sensitive pillow. He found that as eight-week-olds gained contingent control over the increasingly complex aspects of the mobile display, their smiling increased significantly.

Papousek and Papousek (1975) describe the pleasure four-month-old infants derive from discovering contingency relationships.

> . . . as soon as the infant had discovered that light presentation was contingent on his own head movements, his behavior changed dramatically. Orientation reactions increased in intensity, and the infant continuously made all possible types of movements to try to switch on visual stimulation again. If successful, he repeated his feat so many times and with such joyful affect in his gestures and vocalization that it seemed more like attachment than habituation (pp. 251–252).

Papousek and Papousek believe that the actual reward in these experiments is the infant's pleasure in expectation of a response and its confirmation. The discrepancy between expectation and response is both a source of stimulus discrepancy—which leads to learning and schema acquisition—as well as a source of positive affect. Based on their model that the contingency relationship is effective in producing a generalized expectance of control or mastery of helplessness, Lewis and Goldberg (1969) suggest, based on a neurophysiological model, that sensory processing not only involves orientation toward stimuli, but also presupposes an active assimilating of new information.

Further, based on the observational studies of mother-infant interaction, Rubenstein (1967) feels that the quality of the mother's contingent responsiveness to her infant may affect the baby's desire for novelty and familiarity. The mother's contingent responsiveness builds in the infant a sense of security and motivation to produce new behaviors that had not been reinforced in his past experience. He thus acquires new skills.

### Affective Development

There are two major expressions of affect during the first month of life, crying and smiling, which become increasingly elaborated over the infant's first year. Yet in referring to them as affects, adults are inferring the meaning for the baby of the particular behaviors—crying indicates stress and smiling indicates pleasure, for example. Still, the labels provide a guide to the baby's affective states and communicate the adult's emotional response to the baby's behavior.

For the baby there must be a range of internal experience which its cries, coos, and gurgles express, a range that thus far resists measurement and clear adult comprehension. Thus the newborn's cry is usually a sign of distress, calling for the mother to come and feed it, change the diaper, or soothe in some other fashion. But some investigators such as Wolff (1969) speculate as to whether particular patterns of cry correlate with specific messages. Wolff studied types of cries by relating them to the circumstances which elicited them and by sound patterns produced on a spectrograph. In this manner he identified a hunger cry, a pain cry, and a "mad" cry which is a variation of the hunger cry except more turbulent due to excess air forced through the vocal cords. Sander and Julia (1966) measured crying with their continuous automatic monitoring system for infant-caretaker environments, and found that a change in caretakers can result in an increase in newborn crying. Another aspect of crying— unexplained fussiness—becomes prominent during the first two months and declines toward the end of the third month, and appears to be independent of mothering. Two recent longitudinal studies of normal infants (Tennes et al., 1972; Emde et al., 1976) found this fussiness in all their subjects. This is not to be confused with colicky distress that occurs in less than 25 percent of children. The ubiquitous fussiness appeared to have a normative developmental course that was relatively independent of variations in mothering, with an average onset at about three weeks and a decline at three months. Its decline correlated with emergence of the smile in the baby that is provoked by the mother's visage which is a forceful new stimulus eliciting system. The earliest smiles, referred to as endogenous smiles (Spitz, Emde, & Metcalf, 1970; Wolff, 1963), are present in the first week of life. They are mediated by brain stem function, and generally appear when the infant is asleep. The first elicited or exogenous smiles also occur during sleep in the first week, provoked by gentle stimulation of the infant's skin (Sroufe & Waters, 1976).

Slightly later in the second week of life, Wolff (1963) found that elicited smiles occur when the infant is awake following the feed. Typically the baby is glassy-eyed and drowsy, and intense auditory stimulation, especially a high pitched voice, is a powerful elicitor. During the third week, the infant smiles more actively, especially at voices. In the fourth week, the mother's voice becomes an important elicitor of smiling, even causing an interruption of the feeding. By this time, the smile has become almost entirely independent of the baby's state of arousal. Also in the fourth week, visual tracking of an object, such as a hand in front of face, produces a smile of surprise. Seven of Wolff's eight subjects began smiling at pat-a-cake games, and this response remained for approximately three months. In the fifth week, the stimulus value of the voice waned, and the nodding head became the first visual stimulus to consistently elicit smiling. The movement and the configuration of the face provide the complexity that arouses the pleasurable affective response in the baby at this time. According to Sroufe and Waters (1976), the nodding head elicitation of the smile at five weeks is a landmark that reflects the first formation of a true visual schema. From the fifth through the eighth week of life, the infant is most responsive to dynamic visual stimulation. At eight weeks, rotation of a dummy head with blinking lights produces smiling. Increasingly, however, the complexity of visual stimulation alone loses its potency. Like the face, certain stationary visual stimuli become more effective or "meaningful" producers of smiling. Then, from three to five months, as Kagan points out (1971), stimuli such as the face lose their potency to elicit an infant's smile. The baby by this time apparently has a well-articulated cognitive schema of the face. Because the baby readily recognizes the face, there is no excitement or effort required for assimilation of its schema, hence there is a decline in the smile.

With schema formation it is no longer stimulation per se that produces the tension leading to the smile, but the infant's effort in processing stimulus content. Thus, as the infant becomes more actively involved in its transactions with the environment there is no longer a one-to-one correspondence between stimulation and arousal. Also the background stimulation, which the younger infant suppressed or ignored, the older baby can often assimilate as an aspect of the context.

Laughter is another affective response which develops rapidly in the first year. From birth through three months, elicitors of laughter proceed from intrusive stimulation to interesting visual events in a social context. At four months, the "I'm going to get you" game (Stern, 1982) and kissing the baby's stomach produce laughter. At five months, the two games as well as singing "Boom, Boom, Boom" to the child cause gales of laughter. At six months, a rapidly cut off "aaah" sound and tickling under the chin produce laughter. In this manner, from four to six months the level of auditory and tactile intrusiveness required to evoke laughter in the baby declines. At eight months, one-third of Sroufe and Water's (1976) sample laughed at peek-a-boo as well as at approaching objects. Twelve-month-olds laughed at most visual and social items. They also laughed at items which provided the greatest amount of cognitive incongruity, such as the mother walking like a penguin or approaching with a mask. It is important to note that at this phase they laughed in anticipation of mother approaching to tickle their stomach. Further, they laughed when they were given a cloth to stuff into their mothers' mouths. Such a laughter response becomes a product of the cognitively sophisticated active engagement with and creation of novel experiences. Auditory items which swell in sound and then have a sudden cut-off point produce great tension in the baby followed by laughter. The laughter of older infants at the mother sucking on their bottle or walking like a penguin reflects the child's increasingly rapid coordination of schemata and ability to process incongruity.

In summary, smiling and laughter evolve from a response to intrusive stimuli, to a response to stimuli which the child mediates with active attention, to a response to the content of stimuli, and finally towards smiling and laughter that the child brings forth in an active involvement in producing the stimulus itself. Thus emotional expression in infancy derives from the contingency, discrepancy, and context of experience which can lead to strong positive or negative feelings depending on the infant's evaluation of and readiness for incongruity.

## Social Development: The Early Mother-Infant Interaction

The infant's capacity for social interaction with the mother begins at birth and progresses rapidly over the first year of life. The interaction occurs through several sensory modalities: vocalization, vision, touch, hearing, physical proximity. Second, there is a rhythm particular to each mother-infant dyad with a particular pattern of turn-taking. If either partner fails to produce appropriate eliciting stimuli, or fails to respond to the cues communicated, or fails to respond to the other in a reciprocal way, the entire interaction will become dyssynchronous. Organic factors, such as innate differences in newborns (Korner, 1964), may affect the baby's response. Likewise, characteristics that the mother brings to the interaction, such as inexperience, psychological problems related to her own past, or her own temperament in conflict with the baby's (Thomas et al., 1968) may also cause a dyssynchronous interaction.

### Historical Antecedents of the Interactional Paradigm

Speculation as to the nature of the mother-infant relationship began with Freud at the turn of the century (1950). He brought the mother-infant relationship into focus with his concept of the oral libidinal stage of development, and his conceptualization of the impact of oral gratification and frustration in the maternal feeding situation upon subsequent ego development. Despite his focus on feeding, Freud did not delineate the behavioral phenomenology of the mother-infant interaction. Erikson (1950) enlarged the angle of focus to include the mother, child, and social custom in his field. In many respects Erikson was the immediate progenitor of the next theoretical advance which Bowlby (1958) adumbrated with his ethologically based studies of attachment. He brought data from psychoanalytic theory and methodology from ethology and constructed an alternative or complimentary hypothesis to the prevalent drive-reduction views of both learning theory and psychoanalytic theory. According to Bowlby, the infant did not develop a social relationship with the mother out of physiologic need-satisfaction, but out of the innate need for safety through proximity to the mothering figure.

### Attachment and Bonding

Attachment and bonding describe an essential aspect of mother and infant behavior, although the terms are often confused in the literature on mother-infant interaction. Each has a distinct meaning, however. As we have said, attachment refers to the infant's tie to his mother as a proximity and safety-seeking creature. Attachment behavior defines those behaviors which function to maintain the infant's proximity to its mother—sucking, crying, smiling, clinging, following, calling, using the mother as a secure base from which to explore, and greeting and approach behaviors toward the mother after her return from a brief separation (Bowlby, 1969).

Although Bowlby emphasized that attachment behaviors are controlled by a dynamic feedback system between mother and child, the focus was on the child. Attachment behaviors of the child "elicit" maternal caretaking behavior. The equivalent tie of the mother to infant is bonding. According to Campbell and Taylor (1979),

> The term bonding is used most often to refer to a rapid process, occurring immediatly after birth, that reflects mother-to-infant attachment. . . . The quality of bonding is studied by observing affec-

tionate behaviors that the mother shows toward her infant, primarily touching, eye contact, holding, and caressing, which are assumed to reflect that "bond" (p. 3).

It has been argued that the establishment of a close mother-to-infant bond immediately postpartum should facilitate the development of good mother-infant relationships in the first year by sensitizing mothers to their infants' cues. According to Kennell (1974), the postpartum is a sensitive period for the mother in developing feelings of love for her baby. Kennell and his associates suggest from their findings that when the mother and infant are separated after birth and not allowed to be together in close physical proximity, the bonding process may be vulnerable to disturbance resulting in later maternal neglect and/or child psychopathology. Campbell and Taylor (1979) state that bonding is unidirectional—from mother to infant—and occurs rapidly within hours after birth. Thus, this temporal criterion is important; while bonding occurs immediately after birth, attachment continues throughout the child's development. Additionally, writers have often described how the mother's feelings toward her baby begin while the baby is in utero, bringing to bear upon the new relationship the mother's anticipation, affection, fears, and conflicts derived from her personality and her experience with her parents and the baby's father.

Although bonding is unidirectional, from mother to infant, attachment is more interactional. It "develops gradually during the first year of life . . . influenced by such psychological variables as the quality, timing, and pacing of adult-child encounters" (Campbell & Taylor, 1979, p. 3). Ethology typically described these variables as operative in feedback loops. The behaviors are seen as discrete, with initiations and responses, but not necessarily reciprocal. The classical attachment literature (Bowlby, 1958, 1969, 1973, 1979, and revised by Ainsworth, 1978), focuses on the infant's or child's tie to its mother, again not conceptualizing reciprocity. For example, Ainsworth's Strange Situation Test attempts to operationalize the child's attachment to its mother and measure its quality. There are no comparable measures for the mother's behavior in this experimental paradigm.

### The Mother-Infant Interaction: Further Considerations

Call (1964), one of the early researchers in linking attachment concepts with psychoanalytically informed observational studies, delineates an infant behavior which he terms "anticipatory approach." Manifest at feeding, the baby communicates to his mother his wish to be fed with his postural movements. And in their study of the developing maternal sense, Robson and Moss (1970) found that four to six weeks was a transitional period during which mothers become more competent in their caretaking behaviors at the same time that they reported perceiving their infants as being more "human." And shortly later, at seven to nine weeks, the mothers felt their babies reacted differently to them than to other adults and had began to recognize them. As a corollary to this, Emde et al. (1976) found a differential responsivity in the infant in the first two months when the mothers "tuned in" to the baby, that is, when they learned what soothed the infant best and how to time their interventions.

Spitz spoke of the "dialogue" of sequential action-reactor cycles in the framework of the mother-infant relationship:

> By far the most important factor in enabling the child to build gradually a coherent ideational image of his world derives from the reciprocity between mother and child. It is a very special form of interaction creating for the baby an unique world of his own, with its specific emotional climate. It is this action-reaction cycle that enables the baby to transform step-by-step meaningless stimuli into meaningful signals (1965, pp. 44–45).

Further, Schaffer, Collis, and Parsons (1977) speak of dialogue, not maternal monologue, as the basic unit of vocal interchange between mother and infant. It seemed to them that the basic cue for turn-taking in mother-infant interaction was the other partner's silence or inactivity.

The Brazelton group has done a series of important studies of mother-child reciprocity in the first year of the infant's life. (Brazelton et al., 1974; Als et al., 1980). For example, one of their major contributions has been to carefully delineate the concept of "reciprocity," to operationalize it, and to trace its early vicissitudes through empirical studies of analyses of videotapes of mother-infant interactions. Als et al. (1980) define the term well:

> A mutually regulated communication system exists between a mother and her infant . . . serving to meet the biological and psychological needs of both. If either partner fails to produce appropriate eliciting stimuli, fails to respond with appropriate behaviors, or fails to regulate the complementary and synchronous process of his or

her attention or affectivity in the interaction, a nontypical interaction will result (p. 22).

True reciprocity involves a system with input from each partner. The infant can maintain a state in which an interaction can take place; and he has the capacity to be aroused to this state and to attend to his mother, which is important in communicating to her his availability for socializing. On the mother's part, she must perceive her baby's state, alert it with talk, touches, and holding, and facilitate the integration of the baby's actions into ever higher levels of competence.

Als et al. (1980) describe the stages of reciprocity over the first year of life in a blind child and her mother, although emphasizing that the general scheme of this unfolding of reciprocity applies to all dyads. The scheme categorizes layers of infant development:

1. Immobility, the first layer of organization
2. Attentive stillness, the second layer of organization
3. Reciprocity, the third layer of organization
4. The beginning of object manipulation and interaction with other people, the forth layer of organization
5. Infant-initiated interaction with people and objects, the fifth layer of organization

The stage of reciprocity occurs at about three-and-one-half months, which is contemporaneous with the shift from endogenous, or primitive control of behavior to exogenous, or forebrain control of infant behavior. Thus it follows that neurological maturation underlies perceptual development which allows the baby to relate to the mother in a reciprocal way. In order to engage in reciprocal behavior, the baby has achieved at least some capacity to regulate internal states so that it can focus its attention outward, some gross motor control, and the capacity for a sustained interaction with the mother with less alternation of attending and not attending. Further, the baby by this time has a fully developed social smile which is a great pleasure for the mother and strongly arouses her interest and engagement and social interaction.

Dixon et al. (1981) found that mothers display a set of behaviors with their infants which are different from the way other adults behave with the same baby. Mother's first "contain," holding on "to a part of him" to maintain contact, sitting close, using a steady interactional state to focus on the child. The mother's posture, play, expression, baby talk, and dialogue games all speak to her readiness to initiate and maintain interaction. This is qualitatively different from nonparents with a baby, and it seems to function to regulate and increasingly integrate the baby's response systems. Additonally, the steady attention of the mother, expressed through these behaviors, gives the baby a sense that it is being addressed contingently and predictably.

Stern (1971) describes elements of an optimal mother-infant interaction. During the first three months, the mother and infant provide stimuli for each other in which the mother's face and voice are especially important. Arousal and response leads to turn-taking in which basic parameters are the intensity, duration, speed, form, complexity, and frequency of behaviors. He points out that during the three- to six-month period the infant is not just processing stimuli, but actively seeking it. Further, the infant does not orient and remain attentive to any and all stimulation. He is selective in choosing those which are pleasantly arousing. Also, the caretaker who is affectively "alive" (in talking, facial expressiveness, movement, etc.) creates a display that corresponds to those stimuli which the infant prefers. Thus, the affectively available mother is providing her infant with those stimuli to which he is innately attuned, building a synchrony between mother and infant. Stern refers to this as the "dance" between them. Lastly, in a social interaction the mother will seek to maintain the infant in a state of attention and arousal so that it will be able to perform social behaviors such as smiles and vocalizations which please the parent and maintain the interaction. It is noteworthy that this range is different for each dyad. Thus, Stern has analyzed mothers with their twins and found that a mother shares a distinctively different relationship along microkinesic lines with each of her twins as early as the first weeks of life.

### Conclusion

Let us repeat the major observations, and raise some concluding questions about the normative social interaction in the earliest period of life. First, the human infant is born with an extensive repertoire of behaviors. These behaviors make the baby available for social interaction with the caretaker and launch it into the world as an active seeker of stimuli. Second, the mother-infant interaction is contingent on the other's response. The infant is not just a passive recipient of stimuli from the active mother. Third, mother and infant communicate messages long before the appearance of language. This communication is not mystical, but is inherent in the patterns and function of the reciprocity between mother and baby. In addition, major developmental transitions occur between two and three months, based on the underlying rapid maturation of the central nervous system which facilitates communicative modalities.

Our questions about these findings are manifold. What are their implications for pathologic growth? What kind of disturbed dyadic behaviors exist during this earliest period? Is the child especially vulnerable to them during the major periods of maturational shift? How does pathological mother-infant interaction become incorporated into syndromes of illness and the child's personality? How do individual differences in the baby's physiological make-up (thresholds for sensory response, rate of organizational shift, and specific organic defects) affect the dyadic relationship and subsequent psychological growth?

Experience from the Childhood Psychosis Project sheds light on many of these questions in later chapters. But as a precondition for understanding that information, it is necessary first to consider how intrapsychic or psychological structuralization normatively takes place out of the aliment of the mother-infant phenomena of earliest life.

# Chapter 4

## The Internal Mental Development
## of the Infant

In the previous chapter we reviewed the development of the perceptual, cognitive, affective, motor, and social behavioral repertoire of the infant over the first year of life. In this chapter, we consider the contemporaneous evolution of the child's internal mental structures and functions, for which the behavioral repertoire provides observable reference. Inferring mental processes from external reference invites questions as to the internal experience of the infant; how he moves from sensorimotor knowing to representational thought; and how, in interaction with the mother, he develops adaptive self-regulatory capacity. Likewise, it raises the question of how interactional conflict or disturbance with the mother leads to defense reactions and developmental disturbances in the child.

### First Year of Life

According to Stern (1980), the infant's psychic constructs of "self," "other," and various "self-other" experiences may be prestructured—

67

existing from birth as latent, separate entities that result from the design of the human infant's perceptual, cognitive, and motor apparatuses. Still, individual differences in newborns (Korner, 1964) and differences in infant temperament (Thomas et al., 1968) are also important determinants of how an infant will interact with his mother (her own behaviors also modeled by her personality), thus giving a unique quality to each baby's emergent self, other, and self-other mental structures. While the infant has some relatively sophisticated capacities at birth, these will change in terms of behavior and internal mental structures and functions; and we want to look at how the various influences in the infant's life converge and influence his development. The mother's psychology, based on her own identification with her mother and experiences from her childhood, is transmitted to the infant through caretaking behaviors and through unconscious transmission of conflict.

### Internal Mental Development

To begin to answer questions about internal experience and the process of transmission of maternal psychology to the baby, we need to describe seven basic mental structures which exist in the first weeks of life.

*First, the infant has ways of recognizing the array of stimuli—visual, tactile, auditory, kinesthetic, proprioceptive—that result from his own or another's behavior, or from an external or inanimate source* (Pine, 1979). Further, as the infant's schema become elaborated it has the capacity to recognize such sensory experiences as parts of organized wholes rather than unrelated, multisourced, disorganized events. It increasingly experiences stimuli as separate or as integrated phenomena. On an interpersonal level, the infant can communicate preferences to the mother, and through behavior, even from the earliest postuterine days, give her cues as to preferences for stimulation. In terms of development of the visual system, according to Haith (1980), the infant's visual behavior imposes order on its environment, the stimuli in the environment do not impose the order of visual perception.

*Second, the infant has ways of maintaining the integrity of perception of stimuli emanating from one person or thing in the face of competing stimuli from other sources such as its partner, its internal state, or the environment.* Once an infant has integrated a schema, competing stimuli may be familiar, somewhat discrepant, or too discrepant. These different conditions elicit different responses from the infant. Responses range from habituation, attention, shutdown through sleep, surprise, smile, or internal disorganization. Internal sources of stimulation—in particular, distress leading to disorganization—have the power to elicit previous schema for alleviation of the distress. This is more prevalent after two to three months following the shift from endogenous to exogenous control. In normal infants, crying may lead to disorganization, but it does not necessarily alter the baby's internal structure of already accrued schema. By contrast, if the infant cannot obtain a modicum of self-regulation, or if the baby has not experienced continued contingent responsiveness on the part of the caretaker, disorganization could affect mental structures and function.

*Third, social behavior is made up of several behaviors, many of which are performed simultaneously: vocalizations, body movement, and so forth.* The locus of each act and sensory modality is fixed for the infant within certain limits. For example, infants visually orient reflexively to the source of a sound (Brazelton, 1973). By the age of three months, the infant has come to expect that the sound of a voice and a moving mouth should come from the same direction as the visual location of the face (Eisenberg, 1979). The infant's reflexes and expectations influence the integration of two behavioral modalities. It will watch what it listens to and vice versa under most conditions.

*Fourth, the sense of time or rhythm is an organizing structure for the infant.* Many behaviors which are performed simultaneously by one person share a temporal structure. Condon and Ogston (1966) refer to this as self-synchrony: separate body movements must all work together synchronously in the sense that starts, stops, and changes in direction or speed of one muscle group occur synchronously with starts, stops, or changes in other muscle groups. We know this from neuromuscular studies and the microanalyses of films; and the important implication is that each body part traces its own patterns, starts and stops independently, as long as all adhere to a basic temporal structure. This structure assures that changes in one body part occur in synchrony with changes in other body parts. In addition, Condon and Ogston found that these changes in movement occur synchronously with natural speech boundaries at the phonemic level so that "the temporal structure of self-synchronous behavior is like an orchestra where the body is the conductor and the voice the music." Thus all of the stimuli—visual, tactile, auditory—emanating from the self or other share a common temporal structure. The duality of the mother-infant interaction is predicated on this temporal parameter. For the interaction to be synchronous, there must be exquisite timing of mutual cue reading.

*A fifth organizing structure is the infant's matching of the intensity of his behavior in one modality with the intensity of his behavior in another modality, facilitating the early perception of self and other schema.* Termed "intensity contour structure" by Stern (1980), modulations in the intensity gradient of one behavior or modality of behavior will generally match the gradient of intensity of another behavior or modality. For example, the loudness of the baby's vocalization and the speed or forcefulness of its accompanying movement will normally match. As the infant's distress builds, cries crescendo (an acoustic event), leading to the baby's simultaneous proprioception of flailing and sensation in the chest and vocal cords (a physical response). Thus, all of the stimuli in this brief vignette—auditory, tactile, proprioceptive, visual—emanate from the infant and share a common intensity contour structure. Findings from cross-modality studies substantiate the infant's use of common intensity contour structure to discriminate self-schema from other schema. Evidence now suggests that babies are capable of matching the intensity of a stimulus experienced in one sensory modality with the intensity of a stimulus experienced in another modality. Turkewitz et al. (1966) found that infants perceive that the light of a given brightness belongs with a sound of a given loudness. According to Stern (1980), young infants may be particularly sensitive to quantitative variations in stimulation in preference or even to the exclusion of qualitative variations. Therefore, the baby's ability to match intensities across modalities of behavior would be most helpful to it in distinguishing whether a particular stimulus (e.g., the loudness of a vocalization or the speed or forcefulness of a movement) belongs to itself—the baby—or to its mother.

There is significance here for understanding the mental development of the infant and the potential for pathologic derailments. By three to four months, the infant should be able to recognize each participant's behavior in an interaction as having a particular configuration of sensory qualities—i.e., a structure. In this manner, synchronicity, forcefulness of tactile contact, modulation of sound, and array of visual stimuli presented on the part of both mother and infant structure the interaction. Within the bounds of normality, the capacity for cross-modal sensory integration allows the infant to expect the mother's loudness, facial configuration, affective display, touch, and holding all to follow a particular pattern. For example, if the mother's voice is habitually loud and grating, but she is also able to provide soothing in other modalities that is contingently responsive to the baby's discomfort, the infant can match the mother's loudness with her gentle touch, mutual eye gaze, and concerned expression.

The integrative capacity of the infant across sensory modalities allows it to perceive the interaction as synchronous.

However, if the cross-modal sensory communications are uneven, that is, unpredictable in patterning, the infant cannot develop a schema or integrate the differences in modalities. The baby is not able to respond synchronously, and consequently the infant shuts down some of its own perceptual and motor functioning. This serves an adaptive as well as a defensive purpose. For example, by averting eye gaze defensively to avoid the mother's unpredictable visual stimulation and/or forceful handling that is without regular structure, the baby demonstrates the anlage of a sense of self. That the infant's schema are violated carries a threat of cognitive and affective disorganization, and it behaves in such a way as to minimize this danger. Thus presented with a conflictual situation, the infant itself actively avoids it.

*A sixth organizing structure is the infant's capacity for selective visual and auditory attention or inattention.* By perceiving stimulus timing and intensity, the baby can selectively attend the stimuli from the mother or other, and follow it, thus avoiding being disorganized by adventitious sights and sounds. For example, an experiment by Walker et al. (1980) showed how four-month-olds can be inattentive to competing visual events in an organized fashion. Seated in front of a rear projection screen, the babies saw films of different events projected on the same area of the screen, one superimposed on the other. The soundtrack was synchronized to only one of the films. Gradually the two films were separated so that the babies saw the two images on different parts of the screen. Interestingly, the infants behaved as if a film not accompanied by the sound track was a novel event by looking at it more, and they acted as if the film with the synchronized soundtrack was a familiar event by attending to it less. This finding suggests that the baby may be capable of selectively attending to the mother while remaining inattentive to its own behavior, and vice versa, depending on what offers the greatest interest at the moment. By sorting out manifestly complex events in the way demonstrated by the experiment, babies give evidence of a higher level of cognitive processing at four months than was previously believed to exist. The infant can distinguish discrepant from familiar schema and attend to them for a time, sorting out at the same time cross-modal visual and auditory stimuli as in this experiment. We infer that this ability may reinforce the infant's response to the schema of the mother that is emerging at this time, a schema which consists of the baby's percept of the mother's voice and visage. By integrating two schema—the emerging facial percept as a whole, and the older schema of the mother's voice—the baby very early in life begins to discriminate other and mother from self. Infant selectivity and discrimination is part of sensorimotor intelligence as described by Piaget (1937)—the accrual of knowledge through acting in the first year of life.

To reiterate, the infant is active and stimulus-seeking behaviorally. In terms of mental development, the infant appears to be able to perceive that each individual owns his or her own behavior and that the behavior is organized uniquely with regard to time and intensity contour, and the infant can maintain these perceptions in the face of external interfering stimuli. It can also be inferred by two to three months, with the transition from endogenous to exogenous control, that the baby is capable of maintaining these perceptions in the face of moderate internal interfering states such as pain or hunger. If the internal interfering states are not too disorganizing, and the infant has had contingent mothering, the discriminatory structures would remain, although their behavioral functioning may temporarily shut off. In the absence of traumatic interferences, the schema of the principal other—the mother—should remain stable. Moderate changes in maternal facial expression, position of presentation of the face, and voice should not affect the infant's ability to maintain a percept of the mother.

*The seventh emergent structure in the infant, still speculative, is the baby's ability to recognize "causal" relations between itself and its mother.* If the baby can do this, it would be an important initial stage in the infant's early sense of itself as distinct from the other. We adduce the possibility of the infant having this mental ability from demonstrations that infants can be successfully conditioned in the first extrauterine day (Broucek, 1978) and from baby responses that are contingent on the movement of a mobile (Watson, 1972). Further, most things the baby does to itself reinforce the action. For example, in finger sucking, the baby's lip and tongue action exert an increasing pressure on the fingers while they are in the mouth. Similarly, the baby's actions upon others are generally rewarded by an affective response from the person, typically the mother. These are aspects of the phenomenon of contingency discussed in more detail in the last chapter, but it is also likely that the infant gains from these contingent connections its first appreciation of temporal and causal relationships. Watson (1980) himself suggests that three features of causal structure are available to infants by three to four months of age: an appreciation of the temporal relationship between events, an appreciation of sensory relations (i.e., the ability to correlate the intensity or duration of a behavior and its effect), and an appreciation of spatial relations (i.e., taking into account the spatial laws of behavior and the laws of its effects). These three dimensions index a mental structure of causality, according to Watson. They provide the infant with the knowledge to separate the world into self-caused and other-caused effects.

### Object Permanence and Object Constancy

Much semantic confusion surrounds the concepts of object permanence and object constancy. The terms sometimes have been used interchangeably, and at other times have been given multiple definitions, depending upon the particular school of thought. Therefore we shall begin with a brief review of terminology. According to Piaget (1937), *object permanence* refers to the child's awareness that physical, that is to say inanimate, objects maintain their existence in space and time, even when they are not in the perceptual field. The child achieves this in the final stage of the sensorimotor period at approximately eighteen months of age. Cognitive psychologists such as Werner (1937), continuing in the tradition of Piaget, conclude that object permanence depends on the child's capacity for mental representation: the child forms a mental image of the object even when it isn't present.

On the other hand, *object constancy* is a term in the psychoanalytic lexicon. It was first used by Hartmann (1958) to refer to a person (a human object) who exists for the child beyond his need-fulfilling function. He wrote, "This constancy probably presupposes on the side of the ego a certain degree of neutralization of aggressive as well as libidinal energy; and on the other hand it might well be that it promotes neutralization" (p. 163). Thus object constancy refers to the child's gaining the ability to hold a stable image of the human object in mind endowed with modulated emotional investment. According to Fraiberg (1969), "constancy" is employed in the psychoanalytic literature with the specific meaning that a human object preserves its essential character despite the circumstances which surround it, even when highly charged libidinal or aggressive emotions are involved. In their work, Mahler et al. (1975) and Kernberg (1980) have said that object constancy is the end point of true developmental processes. In the first, the child consolidates the "good" and "bad" maternal part objects into a unified whole object who has attributes of goodness and badness. This occurs around the age of twenty-four months; Mahler and her associates (1975) term it "on the way to object constancy." The actual attainment of object constancy occurs at about thirty-six months when the child has sufficiently consolidated the maternal part objects so that they remain stable mental representations even in the absence of mother, and even when there are intense contradictory feelings about the mother. It is concomitant with the achievement of self-other differentiation, according to Mahler. Similarly, Kohut (1971) emphasizes that with self-other differentiation neither absence of the object nor intense affect alter the mental representation of the self or the other.

From this very spartan overview of object constancy and object permanence we move in two directions. We feel that object permanence as elaborated by the cognitive psychologists is a necessary and sufficient condition for the attainment of object constancy, the latter being both a cognitive and affective developmental achievement. Second, since object permanence occurs at about eighteen months and object constancy occurs at about thirty-six months, how does this relate to our current focus on the mental development of the infant during the first year of life? The link to the first year is in the phenomena of the ontogenesis of memory and mental representation. Fraiberg (1969) provides an excellent distinction between two types of memory—recognition memory and evocative memory.

> A memory trace or a mental image of the mother does not in itself imply the capacity to evoke the image of the mother independent of the presenting stimulus of her face or voice. *Recognition* can take place when the person or thing perceived has characteristics or signs which revive mnemonic traces laid down through previous experience. The test for evocative memory is the demonstrated capacity to evoke the image without the presenting stimulus (p. 22).

Mental representation, which develops toward the end of the first year of life and in the second year, thus preceding object constancy, in its psychoanalytic usage refers to the capacity for the mental registering of an image which remains constant and may be evoked without the presence of a stimulus. Memory evocation and registration are built up out of the infant's process of elaborating sensorimotor schema in the first months of life. Stern (1980) makes the distinction between schema representation and mental representation operationally. He states that schema representation cannot undergo the same symbolic transformations that mental representations can; thus, while the baby is continuing to build schema in the first year, it does not have the functional capacity to perform internal mental symbolic transformations of them.

Ironically, seeking to understand the phenomenon of the anxiety that children often experience in the presence of a stranger for the first time at about eight months, Spitz (1957) suggested that it was an indication of object constancy. He writes:

> The child produces first a scanning behavior, namely seeking for the lost love, the mother. . . . The realization that it cannot be re-discovered in the given instance provokes a response of anxiety. . . . The stranger's face is compared to the memory traces of the mother's face and found wanting. This is not the mother, she is still lost. Unpleasure is experienced and manifested (p. 54).

Here we see that Spitz in fact was accurately describing a milestone in memory evocation and the laying down of memory traces which is a way-station in the ontogenesis of object constancy. Kagan et al. (1978) and McCall (1980) have more recently studied separation distress, and they query why the infant cries when the mother is moving away but is still in sight; why the phenomenon is so little independent of cultural differences, such as nuclear family rearing versus day-care rearing which provides the infant with a diverse experience of separation; and why an unfamiliar setting so strongly enhances the affect of distress. To integrate the different aspects of separation anxiety into one developmental explanation, Schaffer et al. (1972) suggest that two processes must come to maturation in order for the infant to manifest such a reaction. The first is that the infant must have an ability to retrieve and hold a schema of past experience, that is, the ability to evoke a representation of the other. The second is that the infant must have the ability to anticipate possible future events. Kagan et al. (1978) elaborate on the baby's disposition to attempt to predict future events and to generate responses to deal with discrepant situations. He states, "If the child cannot generate a prediction or instrumental response he is vulnerable to uncertainty and distress" (1978, p. 110).

Stern (1980), in elaborating on Schaffer's two processes necessary for the separation-anxiety reaction, says that it would be of more heuristic value to divide such reactions into three processes: an improved retrieval memory; an ability to generate expectations of future events; and the ability to generate communicative or instrumental responses to deal with uncertainty or distress caused by incongruities between present events and future representations of events.

Retrieval, or evocative memory, improves greatly at the end of the first year. However there are some findings that demonstrate that some retrieval may be present long before the advent of separation anxiety at eight months. It has been demonstrated that three-month-olds can retrieve with minimal cues the schema of an event that occurred 24 to 42 hours earlier (Watson, 1967; Ungerer, Brody, and Zelazo, 1977). Still, such investigation of early memory relates to the memory of experimental stimuli rather than to the retrieval of memories of maternal or caregiver schema during the first half year of life. However, it is logical that infants would be likely to perform similar recall for their mother. Bell (1970) found recall of inanimate schema to be generalized to recall of the mother in four- to eight-month-old infants. She explained this by the Piagetian concept of "horizontal decalage" which describes the displacement of a mental operation on one class of objects, e.g., inanimate stimuli, to another class of objects, such as salient animate objects, in particular, the mother.

To review the issues relevant to object permanence and object constancy in the first year of life:

1. Recognition memory is present in the infant by six months; a stimulus which revives the schema of the object brings that object into memory. By this time, the baby has a limited retrieval memory which is an earlier developmental correlate of evocative memory. Watson reasons (1967) that if the infant has had positive contingent experiences with an object or person, the retrieval memory capacity is reinforced and thereby increased.

2. Evocative memory is manifest at eight months as shown in the anxiety reaction to separation from the mother. In sum, the mental development of the infant is rapid in the first year of life, with the elaboration of structures and complex functions, eventuating in inanimate object permanence at around eighteen months and human object constancy in the classical psychoanalytic sense at thirty-six months.

### The Mother's Psychology and the Child's Early Mental Development

The infant's first cognitive structure is the schema—the image of an event which retains the properties of the original sensorimotor experience, such as its sound, smell, and kinesthetics. The earliest schema encompass the context in which they are experienced, a context that usually includes the mother. And, a priori, the mother's participation is guided by her individual psychology. Gouin-Decarie (1965) found that the mother is at the intersection of the greatest number of schema for the infant: the mother can be sucked, touched, tasted, smelled, heard, grasped, held, and seen. Because of the endless combination of schema that include the mother as an object, she promotes rapid mental structural development. Out of the interaction between the infant's developing but plastic behavioral and mental apparati and the mother's relatively stable one, the infant's mind becomes elaborated to more complex structural and functional levels.

*The Mother's Individual Psychology*   In outlining parental psychology there are two basic parameters: the impact of the mother's personality on the baby's development, especially in regard to the transmission of her character style, defenses, and conflicts to the infant; and the brief and long-term psychological changes that parents undergo during pregnancy and early parenthood. Bibring (1959, 1961) has described parenthood as a developmental task in which unresolved conflicts in the parents become reactivated at the time of pregnancy and throughout the postpartum. In the process some parents may rework and resolve old emotional issues, their separation from their own parents, for example, and others may continue in a state of maturational crisis. Parents continuing in crisis will often detrimentally affect their own child's development (Ritvo & Solnit, 1957). In extreme situations parents may project their conflicts, reactivated during the pregnancy, onto the infant. The child thus becomes a potential vessel for the embodiment of parental psychopathology. In the typical family there is a middle ground which depends on the presence of mediating variables: healthy as well as neurotically based fantasies are projected onto the baby, and personal growth also occurs in parenthood.

By contrast, where there is severe antecedent psychopathology in the parents the literature suggests that the attendant severe anxiety remains unresolved in parenthood. Anthony (1980) emphasizes that not only are unconscious conflicts, primitive anxieties, and defenses of highly disturbed parents transmitted to the child, but the same parents are likely to create a chaotic home for the child. Troubled parents have the most difficulty as the children pass through the developmental phases which are fixation points for the parents' own disturbances (Anthony & Benedek, 1970). Thus a parent with psychopathology that grows from a disturbance in the earliest developmental stages will have the most difficulty with the child in its infancy. For example, it is not unusual for profoundly depressed parents to be unable to feed their infants because feeding is related to their own unresolved oral conflicts which occurred at the hands of their own parents a generation earlier (Fraiberg et al., 1980). And parents who have experienced traumatic separations from their own parents early in life frequently negotiate their toddlers' tentative movements toward separation by overprotecting them, or, conversely, have a blind spot to their child's insecurities over being apart from the parent.

Other mediating factors in the potential for parental growth during parenthood are the external economic and familial circumstances the parents face. The nature of the parents' relationship and whether or not support is available for the mother is critical. Since the mother has undergone an intense, often disquieting physical and hormonal change during parturition, she needs in her turn the loving assistance of her husband to best respond to the newborn and to allow her to support its complete dependency on her. The mother who is without assistance, the single parent or the rebellious adolescent, for example, often cannot use parenthood as an opportunity for maturation because of the unremitting stress for which there is no help. Success as well as difficulty in child-rearing may also be related to the mother-infant match. Here the temperamental qualities of the newborn play an important role (Thomas & Chess, 1980; Lewis & Rosenblum, 1974). An irritable infant who cries a lot and appears demanding, or an infant who needs constant feeds, may be especially difficult for a passive or dependent parent. In such an instance the mother or father may feel that the baby is depleting his or her well-being, capacities, and emotional reserve. Ultimately the parent may become alienated from the baby.

Perhaps the central mediating factor in child rearing—which radiates its effects to all other areas—is the new parent's relationship with his or her own parents. Becoming a mother or a father heightens the identifications with one's own parents. The unconscious aspects of identification are powerful because parents often unwittingly do to their children what was done to them. For example, in child abuse violent parents, in spite of unconscious beliefs to the contrary, may be identifying with the aggression in their own abusive parent. Thus if a parent's relationship with his or her own parents has been conflictual, that parent is likely to be troubled in certain actions with a child. This trouble then becomes pathogenic for the new generation. Nonetheless, in most families parental identifications are largely positive. The arrival of new children enhances the self-esteem of the mother and father and solidifies the positive identifications with the grandparents. Even where there is intergenerational ambivalence, the new parents often do adapt, do integrate positive and negative feelings, and use normal defense mechanisms such as repression, reaction formation, and altruism to function effectively.

*The Parent's Transmission of Conflict and Its Internalization by the Infant*
As noted, disturbed parents have more difficulty negotiating the psychosocial tasks of parenting, but how does the baby suffer in its own development from the parent's psychopathology? There are undoubtedly many mechanisms, of which several appear in case examples in subsequent chapters. An example from Greenacre, however, (1959) serves as a preface. She describes "focal symbiosis," that is, a fiercely strong interdependence between two people limited to a circumscribed area of the relationship. In the particular context of the mother-infant dyadic "fit," "a peculiar union of the child's special needs and the mother's special sensitivity" may take place (p. 146). She talks about this as a relationship in which there is an area of the mother's pathology that she projects onto the infant or child with intense "focused anxiety or conviction of a corresponding disturbance in the child." In a case example, a mother suffered from a severe fear of going blind and subjected her child to daily eye examinations. The mother's phobia had been dormant until a slight injury to the child reprecipitated it and caused the full intensity of the mother's anxiety to be acted out with the child with little insight on her part as to its pathological nature. The mother's pathologic anxiety focused on the child created a highly charged, highly valued area of interdependence between mother and child, which led to the term "focal symbiosis." The parent's caretaking behaviors with the child were overdetermined in specific ways, and the mother also avoided looking at other aspects of the mother-child interaction, the child's need for autonomy from intrusion, for example.

There are other focal ways in which specific parental anxieties intrude into infant care. A parent with fears of looking has difficulty in maintaining gaze behavior with her baby. A mother with constricted affect has difficulty providing a range of expressions for her baby which are stimuli for mutually pleasurable interactions as well as for the child's development. In this manner, the infant's every sensory modality may be affected by particular behavioral referents of the maternal pathology. Sperling (1982) feels that disturbed mother-child relationships usually manifest themselves in disturbances of the child's physiologic functions. For example, transitory disturbances in sleep, food intake, excretion, and respiration may appear. There continues to be evidence that colic in infants is connected with maternal psychopathology, in particular with high levels of anxiety. If the mother receives successful psychiatric treatment, the infant's colic disappears (Fraiberg, 1981). Sperling further adduces from clinical studies that if the child's disturbances are more than transitory, the parent is acting out or transmitting a destructive but unconscious wish to the child. The transmission of these motives—which Freud (1933) stated were likely to be the wishes on the verge of emerging into consciousness—takes place through some concrete signs which could be received by the child through ordinary sensory perception (Sperling, 1982). The literature on the psychology of pregnancy (Bibring, 1959, 1961; Pines, 1972; Leifer, 1980) emphasizes that during the pregnancy wishes and thoughts which the mother previously kept in check by repression come to the surface. Healthy mothers repress many of these thoughts again following birth; however, in more troubled mothers disturbing ideas may remain conscious. They intrude into the mother's caretaking and her other interactions with her baby, sometimes in a focal manner and sometimes pervasively. The intrusion is not necessarily linear because the unconscious uses its processes of transformation, displacement, condensation, and so on to disguise the actual conflict. For example, a mother's behavior with her infant may mask the conflict and ward off an intention. Thus she may harbor hostile feelings toward her infant and via reaction formation treat him oversolicitously.

Yet even if the behavior of the mother just described was oversolicitous, the very extremity of it would render it nonsynchronous with infant behavior. Likewise, we can speak of lacunae in caretaking when certain actions and perceptions are missing on the part of the caretaker. Winnicott (1965) uses the term "impingement" to refer to the infant's experience of being exposed to a conflicted maternal state. To integrate the concept of impingement into a developmental view of the transmission of maternal conflict, Odgen's view (1978–1979) is helpful.

> In approaching the question of the nature of the process of internalization of maternal pathology from a developmental viewpoint, the discussion must center around the changing pattern of the ways in which the mother and child perceive one another . . . the mother's

role is to be responsive to the infant's emotional and physiological needs . . ." (p. 500).

He presents a case in which the mother could not respond to the infant's needs and was emotionally aloof, forcing the infant to develop autonomous ego functions, such as locomotion, prematurely. The aberrant caretaking and the child's premature accomplishments were the referents of the psychological phenomenon of impingement. "The mother's functioning was not good enough in terms of her ability to remain empathically responsive to her infant in the face of interference arising from her own pathology" (p. 501). One of Ogden's contributions to this literature is his conceptualization of the effects of the maternal pathology on the infant and his speculations about the subjective experience of the infant:

> [The] mother ceased to be a responsively flexible medium and instead reflected the very features of her own internal state. The subjective object was prematurely given definite shape that denied the infant the illusion that she [the infant] herself had created it. This resulted in premature awareness of the separateness of the infant and mother which the infant could not tolerate (p. 501).

He goes on to describe the child's development of a pathological defensive process of identification with the mother in order to avoid the painfully intolerable awareness of her earlier deprivations in care.

Ogden sees the transmission of maternal conflict to the infant as a particular form of internalization. Schafer (1968) defines "internalization" as

> . . . all those processes by which the subject transforms real or imagined regulatory interactions with his environment and real or imagined characteristics of his environment into inner regulators and characteristics (p. 9).

Following this mode, Ogden's case describes a form of internalization that is identification. Through identification with the mother, the child had some capacity for self-regulation. Nonetheless it is fragile because the identification originates as a specific defensive response to maternal impingement. It is the infant's effort to deny the lack of a genuine affective bond between mother and infant.

Ritvo and Solnit (1957) have also reported a clinical longitudinal study of the transmission of conflict which is consistent with Ogden's cases. They found in their patients that the innate characteristics of the infants collided "forcefully with the deepest conflicts in the mother." In normal parent-child dyads, babies begin by imitating parental behavior; as time passes, this transforms into identification. However in Ritvo and Solnit's cases, what the baby imitated was not simply the mother, but the mother in a state of distress in which her psychopathology was most graphically expressed in conflict-laden handling of the child. There subsequently appeared in the children identifications with the mothers' conflicts and distresses which were compromising of normal emotional development but understandable in the context of the babies' lives.

The internalization of parental conflict into the psychological structures of the infant begins with the parent's inability to respond contingently to the baby. The baby in turn develops defensive modes of adaptation to compensate for the lack of aliment from the mother-infant interaction. As time passes, this early disturbance affects numerous psychophysiologic processes.

## Separation and Individuation: Intrapsychic Structure Formation in the Second and Third Years of Life

In this section we consider the intrapsychic structure formation of the normal infant from twelve to thirty-six months. It is important to note that there are several levels to consider in regard to infant mentation. In previous sections of this chapter we most closely examined mental structures and functions of the infant in the first year of life as they were revealed by its extensive behavioral repertoire. Seven organizing structures of the infant's mind were delineated, along with the psychology of how the parent affects the longitudinal internalization of intergenerational conflicts. But in delineating intrapsychic structures, their vicissitudes, and the separation-individuation process (Mahler, 1963, 1965; Mahler et al., 1975), we are at a level of inference a step or more removed from observable behaviors. "Intrapsychic structure" refers to internal mental processes related to ego functioning, the modulation of drives and affects, and the generation of fantasy life, anxiety, and body image. They arise from the earlier formation of schema and representations of the self and the other. They are also intertwined with psychological separation and individuation, which are themselves intertwined. The separation process, occurring at about six months, refers to the child's beginning emotional disengagement from its mother which sets in motion individuation. According to Loewald (1978), individuation is the group of psychic processes in which the "separateness of subject and object as distinct . . . organizations becomes increasingly established" (p. 494).

Mahler postulates four subphases of the separation-individuation phase of development: the differentiation subphase, from approximately five to nine months; the practicing subphase, from nine to about fifteen months; the rapprochement subphase, from fifteen to about twenty-four months; and the development of libidinal object constancy, from twenty-four to thirty-six months. Loewald (1978) reminds us that separation and individuation occur within the mother-infant matrix despite its emphasis on the intrapsychic development of the child. He states,

> Individuation or intrapsychic structure formation is brought about, not by unilateral activities on the part of the infant organism, but by interactions taking place at first within the infant-mother . . . field, and progressively between elements that become more autonomous as differentiating activities within that field progress . . . (p. 494).

### The Differentiation Subphase

According to Mahler, differentiation—the first phase of separation-individuation—is the stage between approximately five and nine months in which babies begin their first tentative steps towards breaking away in a physical sense from the mother. This is commensurate with their new capacities for motility and locomotion. Most infants attempt to venture away from their mothers and stay a short distance apart. Crawling off mother's lap, the baby stays close to her feet. As the phase progresses the infant experiments at greater physical separation from the mother. It develops active pleasure in the use of its own body and the dawning awareness of the separateness of its body from the mother or other persons. The self begins to develop in the form of a body ego, or representation of the body and its intentions, primitive capacities, and feelings.

### The Practicing Subphase

During practicing—the second subphase which spans nine to fifteen months—three important developments occur which contribute to the toddler's growing sense of separateness from the mother. These are the baby's rapid differentiation of its body from that of the mother, with concomitant ego boundary or body-ego formation; the intensification of loving (libidinal) drives toward the mother which, from an interactional perspective, makes the mother's attachment to her child a more specific response to the child's love; and the rapid development of autonomous ego apparati.

The practicing subphase has often been described as one in which junior toddler experiences the world as his or her oyster. This is indexed by expanding locomotor capacities which are used in the service of extensive exploration of the environment. The child is at its zenith, utilizing every sensory and motor modality to take in all the stimulation the environment provides. The junior toddler crawls or walks away from mother with little concern for her whereabouts. Internally, the mental representation of the self and others has neither been firmly differentiated nor established, and therefore the "practicing" toddler does not internally experience the mother's separateness. The child can therefore carry out extensive explorations with the fantasy that self and mother are not quite apart. Therefore mother's whereabouts is no worry. As Mahler puts it, "The toddler seems intoxicated with his own faculties and with the greatness of his own world. Narcissism is at its peak" (Mahler et al., 1975).

McDevitt (1980) comments that practicing toddlers seem to deny feelings of loss or anger brought about by increasing intrapsychic separateness; they seem to maintain the illusion that they and mother are still undifferentiated. This is facilitated by the mother's continued presence and the child's use of transitional objects (Winnicott, 1969) at this time which provide a link between self and not-self.

It is important that during the practicing subphase the toddler be allowed to negotiate separateness at its own rate if normal development is to ensue. Therefore the quality of the mother's attitude towards the autonomy-seeking toddler is important for two reasons. If the mother can support the child both in practicing and in moments of apprehensive need for closeness, the toddler will feel comfortable with its activity and will develop well its autonomous ego capacities such as emotion, thinking, and speech. Second, during this subphase the toddler imitates and internalizes the parents' functioning, whether it be troubled or healthy. The identifications and internalizations of the parents shape the toddler's growing self-representation. The child looks toward other significant people in the environment in such a way as to try to get them to participate in this new found autonomy. With environmental and parental support, the practicing toddler will continue to explore with increasing vigor. Occasionally it will need to check back with its mother for "refueling" (Mahler et al., 1975). Further there may be instances of "imaging" the mother (McDevitt, 1975)—moments when the toddler is so intoxicated by exploration that it becomes momentarily acutely aware of mother's absence or whereabouts, stops its activities, and if mother is not available to touch back to for refueling, may remain immobile, apparently attempting to evoke its newly developing representation of the other, specifically the mother.

By the end of the practicing subphase the toddler has the mental ability to distinguish inner from outer and self from other human objects. It also has the rudiments of a body ego which is based on sensorimotor experiences.

### The Rapprochement Subphase

During the third subphase between fifteen and twenty-four months, rapprochement, the toddler becomes more acutely aware of separateness from the mother. Hence one of the specific qualities of this phase is separation anxiety. The child's former indifference over mother's whereabouts shifts to intense concern. This manifests itself in what Mahler refers to as "darting" and "shadowing" behaviors. Attempting to continue the pleasures of the practicing subphase, the toddler finds that, rather than elation, it brings on anxiety as to the mother's whereabouts. Consequently the child darts to and from the parent. Similarly, when it shadows mother by not letting her out of sight for fear that it will lose her, the child is at the height of separation anxiety. Such behaviors are contemporaneous with rapidly forming distinct mental representations of self and others. Still, the representations have not achieved stability, and the rapprochement toddler is vulnerable to situations in which separation from the parent may threaten the image of the parent and self and create intense anxiety. Further, with the rapid precipitation of mental representation the toddler begins to experience conflict in relation to the mother. He wants to be close to mother to avoid the fear inherent in separation, yet the closeness evokes fears of regression to the prior state of merger with the mother. The child is also conflicted in that it wants to be autonomous, but finds that attempts at independence bring increasing awareness of self as separate and mother as separate. These conflicts at their height, indexed by the darting and shadowing, are known as the rapprochement crisis.

With the resolution of the rapprochement crisis, the child loses its former sense of omnipotence and attribution of omnipotence to its parents. More realistic self-esteem takes its place. Change occurs through a gradual shift on the child's part from functioning that is governed by pleasure and gratification seeking to functioning that is governed more by reality (the shift from the pleasure principal to the reality principal). The child also shifts from primary to secondary process thought. With the resolution of this normative crisis, the maternal images which have been all good or all bad, depending on whether the parent's behavior is gratifying or frustrating at the moment, are unified into a single representation and ambivalence diminishes. The defense of splitting (of the image of the mother into "good" and "bad" to protect the one and the self from the extremes of affect experienced in relation to the other), which had been normative to this point, is replaced by that of repression.

On the other hand, if the rapprochement crisis leads to continued ambivalence and splitting of the object world into good and bad, the maternal representation may be internalized as an unassimilated, hostile, "bad" introject. This outcome is most likely when the love object is disappointing to a degree that reaches traumatic proportions through its being unavailable, excessively unreliable, punishing, or intrusive. The toddler then realizes its separateness too abruptly and too painfully. This results in a too-sudden deflation of his former sense of omnipotence. Thus with such toddlers, the behavioral characteristics of the rapprochement subphase persist. They are apparent in the child's continuing intense separation anxiety, depressive mood, passivity, inhibitions, or in demandingness, coerciveness, envy, and temper outbursts. Psychologically, a fixation point is laid down for subsequent interference with normal development and pathological regressions during stress.

The actual behavior of the parents is very important in the rapprochement subphase because it helps to determine the toddler's evolution of its self-representation which is related to its maternal representation. The toddler assimilates maternal introjects into a self-representation to a significant extent by means of identification. It is this very identification that allows the rapprochement toddler to function to a limited extent independently from the mother (Kohut, 1971). More specifically, it is extremely important for the mother to be lovingly available to the child in this third subphase, for it reduces ambivalence in the child, and interpersonal and intrapsychic conflict. According to Mahler, "It is the mother's love of the toddler and acceptance of his ambivalence that enable the toddler to cathect his self-representation with neutralized energy" (Mahler, 1968), that is, to esteem himself or herself. The relationship with the father is also important during this time. The rapprochement toddler's ambivalence and regressive tendencies relate to the mother, whereas the father typically appears to be experienced by the child as a powerful, "noncontaminated," and helpful ally for identification with and introduction to external reality. The father dilutes conflict in the mother-child relation and helps the toddler move away from regressive tendencies and outward toward autonomous development and individuation. Ultimately, positive identifications with both parents are key elements in the resolution of rapprochement anxiety. The toddler attempts to resolve actual and intrapsychic conflicts between its own wishes and its parents' prohibitions by identifying selectively with each parent.

### The Establishment of Object Constancy

The establishment of object constancy in the third year of life is slow and multidetermined. Its culmination—the capacity to maintain and utilize affectively a mental representation of the loved person—marks the child's ability to modulate emotions and its developmental fusion of libidinal and aggressive drives so that a person can be both liked and disliked. It signifies that there has been significant ego development which subsumes growth of adaptive defense mechanisms and perception and memory.

On the road to libidinal object constancy, the child first gains schema, which are images of external reality and experiences registered on the mind of the younger infant. Then follow representations, which are mental images endowed with fantasies and affect. As we said, by the end of the practicing subphase at fifteen months, the toddler can distinguish inner from outer and self from object, and it has the rudiments of a body ego based on sensorimotor experiences. Shortly afterward, by the end of the rapprochement subphase, the toddler has gained inanimate object permanence and symbolic representation (Piaget, 1952). This combination of developmental achievements marks the full transition from schema mentation to representational thought. An outcome of this is the capacity for mental representations of the self, mother, and self-with-the-other, all of which are endowed with affect. The actual consolidation of these representations takes place over an extended period of time until they achieve the stability of psychic structures at about thirty-six months. With such psychic structures the toddler can perform internal transformational processes, that is, it can maintain an image of the mother and endow that with particular emotions, depending upon its particular internal state and/or external circumstances at the moment. The child can thus alter the affective experiences related to the human object, yet the object also remains relatively invariant in its mind, irrespective of mood, because its basic representation is an outgrowth of past experiences. To have this capacity, the older toddler has attained such ego functions as reality testing, secondary process thinking, and some neutralization and tolerance for frustration, anxiety, and ambivalence.

In terms of the toddler's relationship to the mother in this subphase of libidinal object constancy, the child can tolerate her absences for increasingly long periods of time. When it chooses to play away from mother, it feels it knows her whereabouts and may have thoughts about what she is doing. For example, the busily playing child who is asked where mother is or if she is missed will usually provide a simple answer without needing to seek her out. The actual mother, who earlier in the practicing subphase served as a secure base from which the baby could explore, is now increasingly replaced by the child's secure and stable mental image of her so that it is able to engage in activities independent of the actual mother. At the same time, the toddler is able to have an increased self-awareness of its separateness, and affects of loneliness and helplessness. In this manner, the attainment of object constancy by the thirty-six-month-old has contributed to changes in several spheres of functioning. The child has a greater range of affects and an enhanced sense of well-being and identity, and there is a shift from self-centered behaviors to more mature, ego-determined object relations.

*Conclusion*

In sum, in the past two chapters we have reviewed the infant's progress from a relatively undifferentiated state with the mother to one of gradual differentiation. Each step along the way involves gradual changes and modifications of what is internalized so that higher functioning can occur. Again, using the example of change at the end of eight to twelve weeks of age, the infant who was totally dependent upon the mother internalizes a bit of her functioning in order to be able to have some degree of self-regulation, combined with the capacity to delay slightly the need of gratification. The internalization of mother's rhythms and cycles of responsiveness builds and transmutes very gradually the baby's own psychological functioning. This concept is felicitous in describing transitions in the process of psychic structuralization, and it also suggests ways in which the child slowly replaces the primitive infant-mother self-object with higher order structural functions such as the potential for anticipation and ambivalence which derive from the capacity for self-regulation and self and object constancy.

Our focus has been on normal development in the first year of life, with brief excursions beyond the first year as well as into abnormal development, in order to highlight certain psychological processes. It is often in studying the phenomenology of deviant behavior and growth, however, that we gain a new understanding of previously obscure mechanisms. This has occurred in the Childhood Psychosis Project, and those findings bring further clarity to the developmental interrelationship between inner and outer events, and to the origins of severe psychopathology in young children. The next chapter describes the methodology of the Project per se.

# Chapter 5

# Methodology of the Early Natural History of Childhood Psychosis Project

One frustration in studying childhood psychosis, as well as other forms of severe psychopathology, has been that we have not had visual images of patients' earliest lives and the events surrounding the appearance of the first signs of illness. Our knowledge has been built up from studies of the symptomatology once the illness is established and diagnosed. In addition, understanding has grown from reconstructions of earlier periods in children's and parents' lives through their conscious recollections and through extrapolation to the past from how family members in the present are interacting with each other and with their therapists.

While rewarding, such approaches are also limited by several inbred problems. For instance, parents' recall of their behavior and feelings for a now-sick child during its infancy is often faulty for two reasons: the passage of time has dimmed the memory, and, probably more important, distortion often occurs because of a need to deny or repress painful or ego-alien feelings and memories. For example, a parent's hostility to a child may be unconsciousness, leading to a memory (derived from projection onto the child of parental dislike) that the child never showed affection. Or, by contrast, parents may love a child so well that it has been too painful to acknowledge a defect in a baby until it is recognized by someone outside of the family. Furthermore, pediatricians and other professionals who are frequent sources of early life data are also often unable to see clearly and respond to disturbances in the social behavior of a child or parents because they hope it will pass or they fear to upset the parents. The children themselves are unable to describe their own infancy, of course, since events occurring during the preverbal period of life are likely to have been considerably repressed, and their illnesses have also distorted the children's capacity for verbal expression.

Furthermore, the chronic stress of the childhood psychosis syndrome upon both the family and victim confounds attempts to understand its manifestations once the older child and his parents are in the consulting room or laboratory. The illness has often been present for several years, and a child's chronic withdrawal or aggression is likely to ravage a family so that it is difficult to extrapolate from current emotions and interactions back to what life was like during the child's infancy. Similarly, biochemically based studies have trouble assessing the effects that months and years of severe emotional symptoms may have on a child's physiology.

All of these considerations led us toward methodologies that might bring to life the actual infancy of children suffering early childhood psychosis. One approach is the prospective longitudinal study in which children are followed from birth so that later psychiatric illness might be correlated with infancy qualities and events. However, studies estimate that only two to five children out of every ten thousand develop a childhood psychosis (Hingtgen & Bryson, 1972), and the number of families to study in order to obtain a small sample of children who would succumb to illness would be staggering.

The Childhood Psychosis Project chose an alternate avenue for capturing the infancy of children. This was to gather a series of home-movies that families had made of the infancy of children who subsequently developed one of the childhood psychoses. This approach grew from the need for data about the earliest life of the children, but it crystallized fortuitously when the parents of one of our seriously disturbed children gave us many hundreds of feet of film they had shot of their infant daughter long before they were aware of any difficulties. Our careful review of these films revealed the painful presence of profound symptoms in both mother and child well before twelve months of age, and this set the tone for the initial project and its following ramifications.

Over a period of time, we gathered home movies of infants from more than twenty families with an ill child by approaching therapists treating children suffering an early childhood psychosis and by contacting parents through announcements in newsletters of parents' groups. Likewise, a comparable number of control home movies of the infancies of normal children were obtained through announcements requesting films for a "study of early child development." The children were closely matched for number of first- and second-born, for sex, and for socioeconomic status, with slightly more blue-collar families in the index group than the control group, although the majority of families in both groups were middle or professional class. Both index and control groups were largely of European background, and the parents had been born in the United States. (For different phases of the Project, where indicated, we break down the demographic profile of the families further.)

In addition to the films, the parents of the normal and ill children answered a questionnaire on the children's development and symptoms, if any. We interviewed most of the parents and children first hand, and for the index cases we obtained the children's medical and psychiatric records, which often included verbal or written reports of the psychotherapeutic process.

The infancy movies themselves served as a prospective-like data base for the study of the early natural history of childhood psychosis, providing information that had not been systematically gathered and examined before. The movies showed parents unaware that their babies were unusual or had become sick, and equally unaware of their own disturbed parenting, in some cases, which they captured with their own cameras. The data also confirmed just how vulnerable memory and perception are. This was revealed by many of the cases in our study where movies of the children as infants showed parents who were unaware of specific and tragic problems in the first years of life—their avoidance of gazing at their baby or vice versa, their infant's failure to look or smile at them, and so forth. In some ways even more striking, for nine out of twelve of our children with clear symptoms of illness appearing in their infancy movies before twelve months of age, pediatricians did not diagnose major problems or refer the babies for early psychiatric assessment, and consequently no diagnosis was made until these children were at least three years old. In several of these instances, the pediatricians, nurses, and relatives of the families were succumbing to their own internal wishes not to see or deal with distressing symptoms.

The home-movie data base led to three immediate studies, each with distinct methodologies. The first was a *clinical study of the movies;* the second was the use of judges and a scale to produce *blind ratings of mother-infant interaction* in the index and control movies; and the third was a *Piagetian-based analysis of cognitive development* in the first two years of life in the prepsychotic children.

Here we discuss the methodology of the clinical analysis of the families, the results of which appear in the next chapter. Specifics of the methodology for the other phases of the Project appear with their results in Chapters 7 and 8. At least eight hundred feet of film from the first year of life were used for each case that was studied closely in any phase of the project.

## Methodology of the Clinical Analysis

In the first stage of the clinical analysis, a group of three clinicians who knew the subjects' history viewed the movies of a child in their entirety, alternating between disturbed and normal children. This was a hypothesis-generating period during which we recorded ideas and first impressions. Then followed the application of techniques for the study of nonverbal behavior which had recently been developed by kinesicists (Scheflen, 1972; Birdwhistell, 1970), family-studies specialists (Ferber, 1972), and ethologically influenced researchers (Kendon, 1967; Condon & Sander, 1975; Stern, 1971). These techniques allowed us to obtain a nonholistic but rather microanalytic, very fine-grained identification of the components of behavior which made up the social interactions of the family, especially the mother and baby.

Thus the movies were viewed ten additional times for further impressions as well as for the delineation of a range of key parameters, or categories, of the mother-infant relationship for intensive study. We identified these parameters on the basis of prior theoretical and clinical knowledge, but also on the basis of a growing appreciation of areas of behavior and response that were aberrant in the index movies as compared to control families. In this manner, we decided to focus especially on several categories of individual and interpersonal behavior and clinical pathology. Thus we scrutinized the postural kinesics of mother and child—that is, their rhythm, their use of space, their use of arms, hands, facial expression, affect, posture, body tonus, and physical force. Interactionally, we examined and sought the dyadic patterns of cueing, initiation, responsiveness, maintenance, and termination of social behavior. Also, major modalities of mother-infant bonding appeared in the films as potentially productive of study—feeding, holding (and infant clinging), touching, affective synchrony, vocalization, maintenance of proximity, and gazing. Theoretically, of course, we had been led to the infant's attaching actions by the prior work of Bowlby and Ainsworth. Our own viewing and initial discoveries, however, suggested the importance of also studying the mother's bonding behaviors.

In terms of categories of clinical pathology that could be gleaned in part from the movies, there were the initial signs and symptoms of psychosis, and psychomotor development of the children, and the gross neurologic integrity of the children.

We then sought to resolve subtleties of findings and descriptions in all of these areas with microanalytic techniques. Movies of index and control cases were reexamined one by one. Whenever scenes of one of the above categories appeared, slow motion and frame-by-frame projection was used to study the scene. Members of the research group viewed films independently in this fashion, noting their findings. The team then reconvened to study individual scenes together, arriving at a consensual, largely narrative description of what was evident and transpiring in each family. The next chapter presents these descriptions case-by-case for the first ten families in the project.

## Limitations of the Methodology

Several difficulties were inherent in the family-made home movies. For one thing, the films were not constructed in a standardized fashion, resulting in differing amounts of film for each family and variations in filmed scenes. Nonetheless, over and over families filmed infant birthdays, feeding, bathing, greetings, departures, and play. And embedded in each of these activities were the kinesic, interactional, and symptomatic categories about which we sought information. Thus, although some precision and ease of cross comparison between families was lost, naturalism and new insights were gained.

A further problem arose because families shoot movies periodically, so that we only saw episodes of the children's early life. That is, the movies are discontinuous, and we could not know if a particular parental or child behavior that appeared first at a certain age on film might not have occurred earlier off camera. This limitation is similar to that of cross-sectional types of investigations where one is not privy to events that occur in between samplings. Nonetheless, when a child's symptom, such as hand flapping, appeared on film, this was definitive evidence that it was present by the date of that film. Conversely, when healthy behavior was present in a child, such as responsive gazing and smiling, this too was evidence of the child's capacity at that age, in spite of parental recall to the contrary in some instances. Also, in terms of discontinuity of data we were limited to silent films, the age of sound home movies and video tapes having not yet arrived.

Ascertaining children's ages in the movies was generally easy because the parents usually had dated the films. Sometimes, however, anniversaries such as birthdays, holidays, parental recall, and the investigators' assessments on the basis of motor development led to a judgment of a child's age in particular scenes, and this raised the possibility of some error.

Finally, we had to consider how representative of family behavior were the films. Had the process of home-movie making significantly affected the mother's and child's actions? And, since the scenes were not shot under standardized conditions, could we compare interactional findings in different families? Fortunately, the aforementioned recent work in ethology, family studies, and kinesics has documented the validity and generalizability of the kind of observations the project has made from home movies. For example, Scheflen (1971) has described how nonverbal behavior is both culturally determined and highly individualized; it is repetitively, predictably, and unavoidably embedded in one's responses to social situations. Therefore, the most characteristic kinesics are not materially affected by external events such as a camera recording a scene. Ferber (1972) demonstrated that the greeting behavior of people was not affected by whether they were aware or not aware that they were being filmed. This gives some collateral evidence that what a mother and child do and how they do it while being filmed does illustrate fixed and important attributes of the relationship. Additional evidence comes from firsthand sessions with several of the Project families years after the infancy movies were made. In these cases the family members still showed patterns of mother-child interaction and familial interaction which replicated structurally the film behavior of the infancy period. Further along these lines, the validity of the home movies became clearer when in firsthand contact with some of the families (as therapists or interviewers) we too were drawn into family behavior that had appeared on film months or years earlier. Thus a mother who appeared to avoid her infant daughter's gaze on film also could not make eye contact with her therapists.

Stern's research (1971) is also methodologically supportive of and lends useful correlative information to the Childhood Psychosis Project. He filmed play under standardized conditions between mothers and their normal infant twins. Through frame-by-frame analysis of the eye-gaze interaction of the mother with her twins, he was able to determine that each twin formed a relationship with the mother in which social contact was characterized by a fixed pattern of mutual eye and head movements that differed from the pattern formed by the mother with the other twin.

With this kind of methodological and theoretical background, and stimulated by the provocative, often previously unreported observations the cases were providing, we decided to accept the limitations of our data base—which meant that some of our findings would necessarily be speculative—and proceed with a systematic project. Chapter 6, then, reports the first phase—a series of case studies that integrate the clinical analysis of the film data with the clinical histories of the children.

*Chapter 6*

# Case Studies

---

Case studies often provide a richness of knowledge about families and their members that is not obtainable when a series of patients are studied as a group. By combining information from the analyses of the infancy movies, from the medical records of the children, from the psychiatric case-records of the therapists of the family members, and from firsthand contacts with the children and parents, we arrive at a subtle understanding of the overt behavior and relationships among family members as well as of the unconscious determinants of these behavioral referents and their sequelae. Studying an individual case with the benefit of data from these several vantage points allows us to achieve an unusual synthesis of direct observation of behavior, internal precursors, and clinical findings. Although results from such case studies may not be generalizable as theory, the inferences drawn from them are extremely useful in the generation of hypotheses.

In this chapter we discuss three case histories in great detail and seven more in lesser detail. The first three represent two nosological categories of childhood psychosis—autism and symbiotic psychosis of childhood—as well as three different paradigms of mother-infant interaction. The seven additional cases include the syndrome of Mixed Form of Early Childhood Psychosis, and illustrate further interactional paradigms. The case presentations are organized first with the child's name and the Early Natural History of Childhood Psychosis Project diagnosis for the child.[1] This is arrived at on the basis of case records, interviews with the child and family in some cases, and from the analysis of the symptomatology which appeared on the infancy films. The diagnosis follows the nomenclature set forth in Chapter 2. Then follows a section on the child's and family's clinical history where often appear descriptions of diagnostic labels that had formerly been applied to the children in the course of previous professional and institutional contacts. After this comes the analysis of the film data, and finally a description of the initial signs of illness in the children. Within this organization, each case presentation varies somewhat since the balance of historical, firsthand, and film data for each family was different. The case material led us to emphasize and interpret different aspects of a child's illness in some of the presentations in order to use the available information as fully as possible.

### CASE 1 / Joan: Autism

#### CLINICAL PICTURE

Joan came to treatment when she was three-and-a-half years old, after a nursery-school teacher suggested a psychological evaluation because of her isolation from other children and her lack of speech. She had been enrolled in the nursery school on the advice of her pediatrician, to spur development. The parents themselves had for the first time become concerned about their child's uncommunicativeness and unresponsiveness shortly after Joan's only sibling, a brother, was born when she was three.

When first seen at age three-and-a-half, the child showed many of the classical signs of autism. She spent most of her time by a wall in repetitive, stereotyped activities such as spinning and dropping blocks, sifting sand, or staring out the window. She would also cruise around the room repeating a course that included touching objects and occasionally spinning herself. Not only did Joan not make eye contact with her therapist or parents, she assiduously avoided any eye contact by moving away, or, less frequently, by turning only her head away while remaining near. She gave the appearance of existing in a self-contained world, except for rare instances when she approached

---

[1]Child and family descriptions have been disguised to protect the confidentiality of the subjects.

her mother or father, turning away about three feet before reaching them. She then seemed content to play a stereotyped game close to them. Speech consisted of occasional mumblings, a rare disconnected word or short phase, and rare appropriate words or phases such as "no . . . give me . . . go home." The child's affect was largely one of contented self-absorption. If frustrated or if prompted by internal cues, she might cry piteously. There was no aggressive display. Although she resisted being held, if vigorously swung in the air her initial anxiety often gave way to pleasure or excitement. She was physically attractive. Coordination and locomotion were unremarkable except for episodes when she waved her hands in a flapping motion and her fingers in a dancing motion. These movements or autisms were sometimes accompanied by standing on tiptoes, and frequently occurred when she became excited. Joan had not achieved bowel and bladder control; she used a cup and fed herself with her hands, refusing to eat with utensils.

### DEVELOPMENTAL HISTORY

Joan had experienced a normal pregnancy, delivery, and neonatorium. The milestones of social smiling, sitting, standing, and walking all occurred within normal limits. The parents described their child as always placid and content, making few demands, eating regularly and well, and sleeping easily. The mother breast fed, and by the third month the child gave up her demand for a nighttime feeding and slept through the night. Several events of great significance were telescoped into the fourth month. A great-grandfather, to whom the mother felt a strong attachment, died, leaving the mother depressed and tearful but still pursuing her activities. The father also experienced a family loss. During this time Joan was weaned in a single week because she had begun taking solid food and the mother thought this was an indication to stop breast feeding. In addition, she was moved out of the parents' bedroom. The parents recalled no response from the child to these events.

In retrospect, however, pernicious features began to appear in the second half of the first year. There was no recollection of stranger anxiety then, and subsequently, in the second year, no evidence of separation anxiety when Joan began to wander freely about the back yard and out of her parents' presence even in strange places. When she could stand at nine months, she began a persistent and frequent habit of awakening in the middle of the night and bouncing at her crib rail or sitting and dropping toys while humming or singing nonsense syllables. Later, in the second year, she behaved in this self-involved manner, with a peaceful or serious expression on her face in the company of friends or relatives. The parents felt that she was growing into a very independent, serious girl. At about twelve months, a few words appeared that sometimes seemed to be used appropriately. "Mama" and "Dada" appeared early in the second year, but the parents could not recall with any conviction that the child used these words to identify them. Toilet training was attempted futilely at the beginning of the third year by sitting the child on the potty after meals, but there was no indication that Joan had any recognition of genitalia or other body parts. Her medical history had always been negative. At the time of psychiatric evaluation, neurologic examination, EEG, and other medical screening tests were all normal.

## FAMILY HISTORY

Given Joan's obvious disturbance, it was hard to understand how there had not been a psychological evaluation until she was three-and-a-half. Since the parents were intelligent and not isolated, there must have been a great deal of denial of their child's condition. The father, in his early forties, was an actuary; the mother, in her late thirties at the time of the child's birth, had worked as an accountant before becoming a full-time housewife and mother active in the community. There were several striking features in the histories of both parents. The father was the middle child in a family of several brothers and sisters. A younger sister suffered the first of several schizophrenic decompensations in high school. An older brother and sister were his father's favorites, he felt; they became lawyers. He described his mother as kind, but less influential than his autocratic and self-dramatizing father. As a teenager, he believed that his father belittled him when comparing him to his brothers and sisters. To this he responded by excelling in school, feeling that he could not trust emotions but only intellect. He felt he might hurt himself or others if he became emotional, for he might get too angry. He described himself as consequently shy and was drawn to his wife, when they met in college, by her similar shyness and intellectual interests.

Joan's mother was the oldest of several siblings. Significant in her recollections was the feeling that, in spite of the large family, she was an unwanted pregnancy. She spoke of her mother as overwhelming and intrusive, and had a painful childhood memory of her father taking food from her. She had friends, but felt chronically timid, and the recurrent emotional theme of her life at many stages was that of being used and not supported by her parents, suggesting a paranoid quality. Although Joan's mother was an attractive, well-meaning woman, her actions with her daughter—and with most people—were wooden, mechanical, and uncertain. She had marked difficulty looking people in the eye; she called it her shyness and insecurity, and related it to her battles with her powerful mother. At one level this difficulty suggested strong inhibitions and conflicts about exhibitionism and the visual conveyance or perception of aggression. At another level, there were indications that this represented a more serious fear of and defense against ego dissolution or fusion with another person. Thus, when the therapist left on vacation after a year of treatment of the mother and child, she spoke of fearing death and recalled similar fears in her childhood when people left for short periods. It seemed as if the mother's pathology around the issue of separation paralleled in a less severe way her daughter's failure of individuation.

## FILM ANALYSIS

The family provided approximately 2,000 feet of home movies of Joan which began within hours of the child's birth and terminated when she was three years old, the age she was diagnosed as ill. The movies demonstrated that:

1. On the basis of gross clinical impressions of her physical and motor development, Joan was an intact child without gross neurologic stigmata.

2. The crucial developmental milestones of eye movement, eye focus and fixation, and the social smiling responses were unremarkable until the sixth month.

3. Motor behavior (as demonstrated in general body movement, head and torso control, and manipulation) also appeared normal until the sixth month. Later, major motor milestones such as sitting, crawling, standing, and walking all occurred normally.

4. From birth, the child had less activity, visual pursuit of objects and people, and reaching than normal children have. Such observations were usually made in footage taken when Joan was lying alone in the crib or in the company of toys and family members, and they were compared with later footage of Joan's normal brother, with control films, and with clinical observations of other children.

5. From birth and into early childhood, Joan's body tonus was

more flaccid than is normal. This judgment derived from observation of the child's muscle tension, muscular activity, and posture during periods of rest, quiet activity, vigorous activity, and even pleasurable arousal.

6. For the first six months, Joan's mother repeatedly avoided making eye contact with Joan, although she did look at her child. This is perhaps the most important observation, one which is in the category of social interaction analysis. It requires detailed description to make clear its significance. In one scene when Joan was three months old, the mother forcibly turned the child's head away when she tried to look at her. In another scene at four months (a 30-second episode which was long enough to permit detailed analysis of dyadic gaze behavior between mother and infant), the mother repeatedly avoided making eye contact with the baby. Her eye and postural behavior was dyssynchronous with the child's, so that she removed her head from the baby's field of vision when the baby turned to her mother. Figure 6-1 through 6-4 are sequential drawings of this interaction. A composite of the sequence, the figures cannot detail every movement since they cannot reproduce all of the steps that the frame-by-frame analysis of the film reveals. The full sequence is described below, illustrated by the drawings that most closely depict each phase of the interaction.

At the beginning of the sequence the child is being held by the mother (Figure 6-1). Both child and mother appear relaxed and content. At first smiling, the child then turns both head and eyes toward her mother's face. The mother's expression becomes tense; and as she tenses instead of turning to her child, the baby also loses her smile (Figure 6-2). The mother then (Figure 6-3) inclines her head backwards and to the side of the child's face so that the child's head is blocked. The baby cannot turn her head further to bring herself face-to-face with her mother; the child's eyes are to the right as far as she can turn them, but she cannot reach her mother's face or eyes with her own. The baby's affect in quick succession becomes tense, then desperate, then dejected. Finally (Figure 6-3), the child has given up trying to turn to her mother, and the mother herself is more relaxed (Figure 6-3), the evasive actions having been successful. The mother and baby then (Figure 6-4) resume the same postures as in the beginning of the sequence, although the child's affect is initially depressed in reverting to this position. At this point (Figure 6-4), the mother begins to caress her daughter's head; the baby drools slightly with pleasure and begins to smile. This completes the sequence of illustrations. At this point in the movies, however, the whole interactional sequence repeats itself when the child again attempts to look at her mother.

Rare scenes did appear when the mother met Joan's gaze. However, she was at arm's reach from the baby and outside of the child's best focal distance. On one occasion, the mother met her daughter's gaze while a relative held her. She held this position for a moment before placing her face directly in contact with the child's. This also effectively blocked dyadic gaze. That this behavior was strikingly aberrant is confirmed by comparison to control films, as well as to later scenes with the younger, healthy sibling. There are many scenes in which the mother fixes her gaze on the younger sibling's face while holding the baby comfortably in her arms.

Further interactional analysis of Case 1 revealed that from the baby's first month, the mother rarely initiated activity that might arouse a response in the baby. The mother was stiff and self-contained: the movies captured no cuddling or playfulness. On the other hand, the child actively initiated contact with her mother in the first half year.

## INITIAL SIGNS OF ILLNESS

Symptoms of childhood psychosis first appeared on film when Joan reached her sixth month. Starting about this time, the child no longer initiated eye contact with her mother, and since she no longer looked at her, she lost visual pursuit of her mother at close or long range. In her sixth, seventh, and eighth months, her expression became more and more self-absorbed and her affect more and more constricted, showing little pleasure or displeasure. By the ninth month, she began to have episodes of what appeared to be hallucinatory excitement—a response not to people or things in her environment, but to some internal stimulus. She also began to show intense pleasure in accompaniment with her increasing ability at locomotion. By the ninth month, Joan had fixed psychotic behavior. She kept physical distance from people and looked only at objects. Moreover, she had developed peculiar shaking and rotating movements of her hands and dancing movements of her fingers, as if she were playing an imaginary piano. These autisms appeared frequently and lasted for a few seconds, often when she was excited, often for no apparent reason.

Although symptoms were not apparent until six months, Joan may have had prodromal signs of childhood psychosis as early as the first three months. Prodromal signs in the first three months, for example,

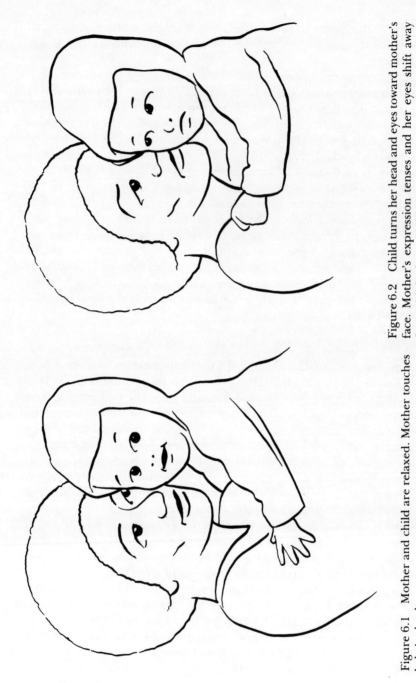

Figure 6.1 Mother and child are relaxed. Mother touches baby's cheek.

Figure 6.2 Child turns her head and eyes toward mother's face. Mother's expression tenses and her eyes shift away from child's face. Child tenses.

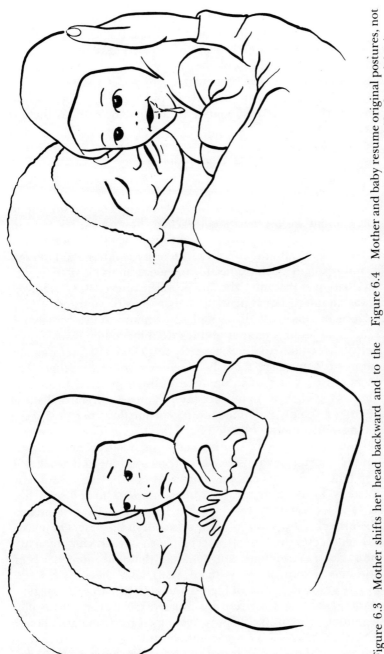

Figure 6.3 Mother shifts her head backward and to the side of child's face, blocking child's facial approach and obstructing eye contact. Mother relaxes. Child appears dejected.

Figure 6.4 Mother and baby resume original postures, not in eye contact. Child's expression shifts from dejection to pleasure and drooling appears when mother pats child's head.

may have been her less-than-normal activity, visual pursuit, and reaching, and her flaccid body tonus. Prodromal signs in the second three months may have been her lack of attentiveness to, fixation on, and excitement at people or objects.

Table 6-1 summarizes the film analysis of Case 1, and serves as an overview of the case, giving a chronologic picture of the mother-child relationship, the longitudinal course of key behaviors, and the appearance of symptoms.

## CASE 2 / Tony: Autism

### CLINICAL PICTURE

The oldest child in a family of three children, Tony first came to psychiatric attention just before he reached three years. His parents felt he was too aggressive with his infant brother, born when he was one-and-a-half. He also did not play with other children, had too few words, and responded unpredictably or not at all to his parents.

On evaluation at that time, the only word he uttered was "bye-bye." There was no interactional play; his activity mostly consisted of handling objects or randomly throwing balls. There was eye contact between the child and his mother and his examiners, but it was unpredictable. So was interpersonal contact, the child only occasionally responding to a message from his examiners or his mother. The examiners sensed a lack of recognition in his seeming not to notice when he was spoken to or approached. Tony was retarded in all parameters of motor and fine-motor coordination, personal-social functioning, and adaptive functioning. The child guidance clinic that saw him found no evidence of organicity, suspected mental retardation, but did not rule out autism. When Tony was four-and-a-half, the family sought further evaluation. Tony was now having severe temper tantrums, in which he thrashed till exhausted, hit and scratched himself, and occasionally cried out "help, help." These tantrums might be provoked by frustrations or arise out of the blue. On intake, he was diagnosed as suffering from a psychosis of early childhood of a form most closely resembling autism. Since that time Tony has been in continuous treatment. Now, many years later, he is in his age-appropriate grade in a normal high school. His intellectual functioning is average, although he remains isolated from peers and is only now beginning to express affiliative feelings for classmates. Though the bizarre behavior of his early childhood is long past, he maintains rigid obsessive habits, and therapeutic content includes such borderline phenomena as occasional confusion of ego boundaries. There have never been hallucinations.

## DEVELOPMENTAL HISTORY

At the time of intake, the parents revealed that they had been concerned about their child's lack of responsiveness when he was as young as six months. They had not mentioned their concern until he was three for fear that they were worrying too much, and because the family pediatrician said that he was a healthy child. Only in the second year were the parents convinced he recognized them. He was two before he said "mama" and "dada." Further developmental history revealed that the first six months of Tony's gestation were complicated by hyperemesis. At birth the child was slightly cyanotic and icteric, and therefore was kept in an incubator for the first two days. Otherwise, his medical history has been negative, as have been EEG and appropriate neurologic tests.

The child is reported to have smiled at three weeks. He was switched from breast to bottle feeding at four months without observed reaction, the mother reported, because she had a sinus infection. In the first six to twelve months, the parents remarked that he "seemed to need no one." Sitting, crawling, standing, and walking took place normally. At seven months, a stereotyped mannerism was noticed. When puzzled or when reaching for an object beyond his grasp, Tony squinted and then began rhythmically to clench and unclench a hand. When he began to walk at the end of his first year, the hand movements changed to a waving, flapping motion, accompanied by dancing, athetotic-like motions of his fingers similar to those described in Case 1. He also frequently walked on tiptoes when excited, and at other times he had a stiff, broad-based gait. These mannerisms persisted well into his middle childhood.

When he was sixteen months old and his brother was born, his mother weaned him from the bottle. She observed that he ignored his brother at first, but his vocalizations became angry in tone. At twenty-one months, when the infant brother was moved to his room, the temper tantrums began. At two years there appeared transient phobias of slides, swings, and rocking horses. With the birth of a second sibling, a sister, when he was three years, Tony developed periods of severe constipation. At the same time he first began using the toilet for urination. His mother, lackadaisically, and his father, angrily, had been attempting to toilet-train him since he had been eighteen months. But at three-and-a-half, when his parents divorced,

**TABLE 6-1** Summary of film observation in Case 1 (Joan). The observations comprise a chronological picture of the mother-infant interaction, child's earliest signs of illness, and child's physical development

| Age in Months | 0–3 | 3–6 | 6–9 | 9–12 | 12–15 | 15–18 | 18–21 |
|---|---|---|---|---|---|---|---|
| Dyadic gaze between mother and infant | C. attentive to M.<br><br>M. does not look at C. | C. attempts eye contact with M.<br><br>M. avoids C.'s eyes and blocks C.'s facial approach. | C. no longer looking at or attempting eye contact with M. | C. selectively avoids M.'s looks.<br><br>M. now begins to look briefly at C. | | | |
| Mood of infant and mother | C. content, has prominent social smile.<br><br>M. has fixed smile throughout first two years. | C. dejected when blocked from seeing M.'s face.<br><br>C. generally irritable. | C. increasingly self-absorbed; little affect except pleasure with locomotion. | | | | |

| Category | | | | |
|---|---|---|---|---|
| Initiation of activity and responsiveness of mother and infant | M. wooden; no initiation of cuddling or playfulness. | M. places C. in "double bind."—M. pats C., C. smiles and tries to look at M., M. pulls away, C. is dejected and gives up; M. then repeats sequence. | C. ceases to attempt eye or body contact | C. looks only at inanimate objects. C. keeps distance from people. Parents attempting contact with C. |
| Signs and symptoms of childhood psychosis | | Lack of attentiveness, fixation, or excitement at people or objects. | No visual pursuit. No eye contact. Self-absorbed. | Stereotypic hand and finger motions. Looks only at objects, keeps distance from people. Hallucinatory, internal excitement. |
| Atypical or delayed development | Less than normal activity, visual pursuit, and reaching. Flaccid body tonus. | | | |

NOTE: Table 6-1 data from film analysis of Case 1. Age of child in months shown horizontally. General categories of observation shown vertically in left column.
C. refers to child. M. refers to mother.

Tony lost his bladder training and began to urinate on the bed, sofa, and rugs. Ironically, however, he deposited his bowel movements for the first time in the toilet, although periods of constipation and soiling also continued.

## FAMILY HISTORY

Tony's mother and father met and married in graduate school, and Tony was born two years later. The mother's appearance and manner were plain and unassuming, and she was reserved, seclusive, and passive. She saw a likeness between herself and her father, whom she described with distaste as cool and distant. She "never knew what he felt," for he showed strong feelings only about abstractions like politics. She said she feared her son's anger, responding to it with rage or withdrawal. Her mother, she said, had a more outgoing veneer, but hid her feelings too. Her childhood family read much and interacted little, either among themselves or with people outside, a pattern she continued in her adult years. She said that she felt that all she liked was fantasy and that she didn't like real people around. Although trained as a teacher, she feared being unable to control a class.

The father, on the other hand, was more outgoing and very self-assured. He needed to be in charge. Early in the marriage he proved a better cook than his wife—a source of mutual irritation, and just one example of the many conflicts between the husband and wife.

## FILM ANALYSIS

There were approximately 1,400 feet of home movies of the child's life from two months to three years. Although analysis of these films reveals similarities with Case 1, there were significant differences between the course of Tony's physical and interactional development, on the one hand, and that of Joan and of normal controls, on the other. Analysis of the films demonstrated that:

1. Like Joan, Tony was born without gross neurological stigmata.

2. Tony did have a social smiling response within the first three months, but it was lifeless and placid. In later months, his smile never conveyed excitement or recognition in response to his mother's face or presence. Contrast this with the pleasure Joan showed and the vigorous attempts she made to look at her mother in her first five months.

3. Eye movement, focus, and fixation were present at their expected times.

4. A notable delay in motor development appeared between five and six months. When pulled from a supine to sitting position, the child's head lagged backwards; and even when sitting, he was unable to hold his head erect and steady. Likewise, between three and six months the child showed no anticipatory adjustment to being lifted by his parents. Otherwise, general body movement, head and torso control, and manipulation progressed within normal limits. In addition, later major motor milestones occurred normally.

5. From birth, the child had a flaccid body tonus. Throughout most of his first year, he had less-than-normal activity, reaching, visual pursuit, and attention to and excitement at objects and people. These observations are like those made of Joan's infancy, but in Tony's case they are more striking.

6. In the category of dyadic gaze behavior between mother and child, from two to six months of age there were numerous scenes in which Tony looked briefly (1 to 5 seconds) at his mother, who did meet his gaze. Tony would then break eye contact by looking away. On the other hand, if the mother looked at Tony, he did not meet her gaze unless she was also physically stimulating him. He might then look at her face briefly before breaking eye contact. By seven months, Tony made only rare, fleeting eye contact with his mother or father. By this time, the mother and father had markedly stepped up their attempts to elicit a look or smile from their child by increased touching, holding, and looking.

7. Tony's mother was like Joan's in being stiff and self-contained. She did not spontaneously initiate cuddling, show playfulness, or mold herself to her child. At five months, an impressive interactional behavior appeared for the first time, and it was to reappear frequently, characterizing Tony's relationship to his mother. While his mother held him, Tony tried to struggle away. Before this, the child had shown no sign of molding. After this, body contact aroused in him obvious displeasure and an attempt to create distance unless he was being forcefully stimulated with motion—as when his father swung him aloft, for example. Throughout his infancy and early childhood, Tony showed no displeasure at loss of eye or body contact. At about six months, when the parents began actively to attempt social games, Tony would not play.

8. Mood and expression were similar to those of Case 1. During the first three months, the child appeared largely placid and contented and the mother's mood was also placid and self-contained. Between three and six months, the child's placidity gave way to irritability and

apparent depression. After that, Tony's affect constricted. After six months, he rarely showed pleasure or displeasure. At the same time, depression first appeared in the mother. The final mood change occurred when Tony gained locomotion. With crawling and especially with walking, his mood improved tremendously and he showed great pleasure. Toward one year of age, his principal expression was one of great self-absorption.

### INITIAL SIGNS OF ILLNESS

Tony's first sign of childhood psychosis may have appeared at three months. He had a peculiar squint when he looked at people and objects. At the end of his first year, it became so marked it could be called a habit disorder. As the squint worsened at one year, a prominent hand-flapping stereotypie appeared.

What may have been other early signs of impending psychosis appeared between three and six months: lack of attentiveness to and excitement at objects and people; lack of molding to his mother; and lack of visual pursuit of or fixation on people or objects. By six months, clear symptoms of childhood psychosis were present: active avoidance of physical contact with his mother; absence of social interaction with his parents; and absence of affective contact with people.

### CASE 3 / Amy: Symbiotic Psychosis of Childhood

### CLINICAL PICTURE

Amy was the first child born to Mr. and Mrs. S. Her psychiatric history began when she entered nursery school at age four. For the first four months of nursery school she did not allow her mother to leave. She would lie on the floor screaming in terror and helplessness—only rarely with anger—and ultimately regress to thumb-sucking and autistic states. Also present at that time were a very short attention span, twisting and writhing movements of the fingers, fear of touching toys and sitting on her buttocks, and a stiff, rigid walk. Speech fluctuated, but there was occasional clarity and pronominal and syntactical correctness. Shortly after this, she began intensive treatment. By her fifth year, Amy repeatedly took the role of provocateur and victim with peers in her day program, where she was diagnosed as suffering a symbiotic psychosis of childhood. A year later, at age six, verbal relating had developed in addition to the nonverbal behaviors. At this time, a paradigmatic experience occurred between mother and daughter at her treatment center. Amy asked her mother where the elevator was. This was a nonsensical question, as Amy knew that the treatment center had only one story. Anxious to relate and fearful of disappointing her daughter, the mother suggested they look for it and find out if there was an elevator. The girl's questions became more and more confused and driven. The mother became flustered and tense and was unable to give a serious answer. This was a typical example of the family's mode of relating: anxious ambivalence over mutual responsiveness, closeness (gratification), and autonomy (frustration) led to a stubborn, teasing, and defiant game that involved everybody in confused expectations. In this instance with the illusory elevator, Amy and her mother became helpless and frustrated, unable to resolve the problem and reduce their tension.

A further illustration of the ontogenetic course of Amy's behavior occurred in treatment at seven years of age. At lunch with her therapist, Amy first took the food the therapist gave her and then spit it out, saying it was sour. Nor would she eat the lunch her mother had sent with her. Similarly, she had not used the toilet at school. She remained intensely fearful of taking things (food) inside of her and of letting things (feces) go. It seems that she was paralyzed by the countervailing forces of her greediness on the one hand, and fearfulness on the other hand, in her cathexis to both people and her own body. In her fantasies in her sixth and seventh years, she repeatedly spoke of cities populated by dead people. She sometimes played that she was either in or causing an earthquake, then lost touch with reality and became terrified that an earthquake had occurred.

## DEVELOPMENTAL HISTORY

Amy's pregnancy and neonatorium had been without problems. Neuromuscular milestones were unremarkable. But from birth the parents said that the child was unduly irritable and sensitive to such things as wind, which caused her to cry. In retrospect, the parents recalled bizarre mannerisms, tantrums, and autistic states from age three. Also the mother recalled at least a year of clinging prior to this. However, the first behavior that had actually consciously concerned the parents was Amy's provocative testing in her third year. These were largely nonverbal interactions in which the child repeatedly attempted to do something she was not supposed to do and was repeatedly stopped. Shortly afterward, in the first months of nursery school, Amy couldn't allow separation from her mother. The threat

**TABLE 6-2** Summary of film observations in Case 2 (Tony). The observations comprise a chronological picture of the mother-infant interaction, child's earliest signs of illness, and child's physical development

| Age in Months | 0–3 | 3–6 | 6–9 | 9–12 | 12–15 | 15–18 | 18–21 |
|---|---|---|---|---|---|---|---|
| Dyadic gaze between mother and infant | C. makes brief eye contact with M. who responds. C. breaks eye contact. | | C. makes only rare, fleeting eye contact. | | | | |
| Mood of infant and mother | C. placid, content, has social smile. M. placid, content. | C. irritable, depressed, but shows no displeasure at loss of contact with M. | C.'s affect constricted; rarely shows pleasure or displeasure. M. depressed. | C. shows great pleasure with locomotion. | C. has self-absorbed smile. C.'s facial expression strikingly pinched and determined with eyes squinted. | | |
| Initiation of activity and responsiveness of mother and infant | M. stiff, self-contained; does not initiate cuddling or playfulness. | C. pulls away from M. and does not mold. M. can elicit look from C. only with physical stimulus. | C. has no displeasure at loss of body or eye contact; does not engage in social games. | M. and father not able to elicit look or smile from C. by touching, holding, or looking at C. | | | |

| | | | | | | |
|---|---|---|---|---|---|---|
| Signs and symptoms of childhood psychosis | Squints at lights and when looking at people or objects | Lacks attention and excitement at objects and people. Pulls away from M., no molding. | No visual pursuit or fixation. | Self-absorption. Active avoidance of body contact with M. Stereotypic hand motions. | No response to people, pets, and toys. | Prominent stereotypic hand-flapping and eye-squinting. |
| Atypical or delayed development | Flaccid body tonus. Diminished activity, reaching, and visual pursuit. | Head falls back when pulled to sitting. Lack of anticipatory posturing when lifted. | | | | |

NOTE: Table 6-2 data from film analysis of Case 2. Age of child in months shown horizontally. General categories of observation shown vertically in left column.
C. refers to child. M. refers to mother.

117

of separation reduced her to helplessness, which paradoxically made the little girl powerful as she immobilized her mother and the nursery school staff. Thus Amy could neither experience autonomy nor allow autonomy in others.

These examples of typical behavior and psychological states observed by therapists and recounted by the parents provide a longitudinal view of Amy's growth. Their potential links to the environment of her infancy become clearer in the family history and the home movie analysis which follow.

## FAMILY HISTORY

The oldest child in a working-class family, Amy's mother recalled her childhood as filled with confusion and anxiety. Her father's inability to separate from his mother led to a chronic unhappiness in her parents' marriage. When, at her mother's insistence, her parents finally moved away from her father's mother, the grandmother died shortly afterward. From this and other experiences, both of the mother's parents conveyed to her that separation and self-assertion were harbingers of destruction. In addition, both parents were largely unavailable to Amy's mother—her father because of his continual depression and overuse of alcohol, her mother because she displaced much of her anger at her husband onto her daughter.

In her teens and twenties, Amy's mother felt inadequate, different, and isolated from peers. Unable to separate from her parents, she dropped out of college and began to work effectively as a clerk, which she continued to do until her daughter was born. In her own marriage, the mother replicated her mother's plight; Amy's father was not able to leave his mother who lived with the family.

Amy's mother's real emotional investment in the marriage was her anger and helplessness in the face of her mother-in-law. But, because she feared her own destructiveness as well as identifying masochistically with her father's incompetence, Amy's mother could not assert herself and act independently of her mother-in-law. She would rush to cook a second dinner for Amy if the mother-in-law criticized the first. Such criticism was an example of the charges of incompetence leveled by the mother-in-law. Needless to say, the father was unable to support his wife. Similarly, when Amy was troubled in her sleep at about one year, her mother would spend the night in a chair with the child draped over her shoulder rather than "risk" putting her to bed again and hearing her cries.

In this context of social isolation, frustration, and anxiety over feelings of inadequacy, the mother's symbiotic relationship with Amy began—when Amy was one year old, the mother spent many nights sitting in a chair with the child draped over her shoulder. She carried Amy in her arms while vacuuming, which was both uncomfortable for the mother and entrapping for the daughter. Their symbiosis was predicated largely on the mother's need to protect the child from her own felt badness and destructiveness.

Diagnosis of the mother must reflect the great unevenness of functioning, from effectiveness to incompetence. Her major conflicts seemed to be oedipal. Themes of guilt and punishment underlay her anxiety and motivated her actions. In addition, earlier developmental issues had been inadequately resolved. Her inability to set limits and to establish effective boundaries between herself, her child, and her mother-in-law suggested an irresolution of issues of control and autonomy. Occasionally, her passivity was interspersed with such aggressive outbursts as throwing Amy in the bathtub with her clothes on in response to her negative behavior. The mother's difficulty with modulating angry expression suggested more primitive functioning. Though the mother was often aware of her feelings and of reality, under stress her behavior and her inner and outer perceptions were distorted by denial, projection, and intellectualization.

The father's background was also replete with psychological chaos. At age two-and-a-half he lost his own father. During the father's boyhood, there was further family disruption. He had little access to his mother who worked six days a week, twelve hours a day. For a time he had to live in foster homes, and from this period he dated his sense of intellectual and social inadequacy. With peers, he began to feel awkward. With his mother, he was hostile and dependent, blaming and tormenting her for his failings. Amy's father lived at home with his mother while studying dentistry; after marriage, the mother joined the new couple. After two years their daughter, Amy, was born.

Though he married and achieved competence in work, his mother's view of him as helpless continued to be the father's own self-image. For example, when the father was asked if he could really pay his bills if his mother did not remind him, he was not sure. He expressed in treatment the view that his child was always on the edge of extinction from starvation or a cough or unhappiness or a crying spell. Any demand or limit-setting would catapult his child into such feelings of rejection that she would not recover from being unloved.

The father was unable to separate his daughter's needs and feelings from his own sense of having been abandoned. He identified with both his child as victim and his mother as perpetrator. Thus immobilized as a parent through his belief in his daughter's vulnerability and his power to destroy, he directed his aggression at his wife. In this manner, he was an extension of his mother, disparaging his wife and further compromising her ability to mother.

## FILM ANALYSIS

The family supplied 900 feet of film of the first three years of Amy's life. Just as the therapists had observed the girl's movement and interaction with her mother and others, so also the movies revealed patterns of infantile behavior and mother-infant interaction. These patterns characterized the relationship from the initial weeks. As time went on and motor development became more complex, the behaviors likewise became more elaborate. Yet the prototypical interactions of the earliest months remained embedded in the later activities, several of which have already been described in the child's and parents' histories and in observations during therapy.

The principal film analysis findings are listed below:

1. Amy's neuromuscular development and her constitutional integrity as reflected in her relative vigor and activity were assessed as follows: Neuromuscular development was normal in the first two years, on the basis of film observation. Constitutionally, the child in her first three months appeared more somnolent, to have a lower level of activity and attentiveness, and to have a slightly more flaccid body tone than control children. After three months these differences disappeared.

2. In the first scene of the mother holding her child at one month, the mother's arm straps the baby against her chest, the seat supported slightly on her hip (Figure 6-5). Holding is so tight that the child is allowed no free movement. The child hangs limply against her mother's arm and body restraints. This position recurs several times in films of the child's first half year. In behavioral terms, though closeness is permitted, it does not allow reciprocal interaction by mother or child in the direction of typical human species ventral-ventral attachment.

3. In the first spoon-feeding scene at one-and-a-half months, the child lies across the mother's knees at a considerable (and abnormal) distance from her torso. Feeding takes place mechanically between spoon and mouth, with no participation of either mother's or child's body. This scene recalls Harlow and Harlow's (1956) experimental

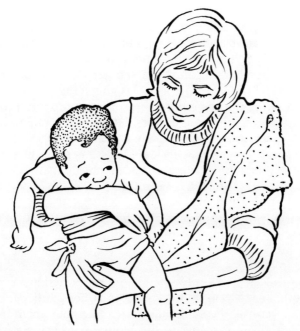

Figure 6.5  1 month. Mother holds child with chest turned away, and rigidly immobilizes baby's torso to her by strapping her right arm around baby's midsection. Baby is not supported from below and hangs limply and apathetically.

nursing situation with monkeys. When they were given bottles on wire frames, this maternal deprivation proved to have psychological consequences, akin to psychosis, far more severe than those suffered by monkeys allowed to have cloth surrogate mothers. As Amy's feeding progresses, she drops off to sleep. Unaware, the mother continues for some time to insert the spoon into the mouth of the sleeping child. She flails back at the mother and spoon, and turns her head away in a stuporous manner.

4. In the first breast-feeding scene when Amy is one-and-a-half months, the baby is closer to the mother's chest and better supported. She is alert and a smile appears. As breast-feeding ends, the baby rotates more and strains toward the mother. She is gazing intently at her mother's face, and the mother smiles fondly in return. However, the mother's torso remains inflexible, with no segmental movements, as if ensconced in armor. In contrast to mothers in control movies, there is no reciprocal inclination of any segment of her body toward the child. The mother's hand hangs limply at the child's side.

5. At two months, the mother holds the child to her in the ventral-ventral position. Nonetheless, full chest-to-chest contact is minimal, for the mother never supports the child around the back in such a way as to bring her into full opposition, and, after a few moments, the child throws her body against the mother. Meanwhile, the baby's hands in normal fashion have been clasping at the mother's blouse to attach themselves, but she is not given sufficient support. Close observation indicates that the mother does not nuzzle the child with cheek-to-cheek contact (as we see routinely in control movies) though only an inch separates them. In effect, full attachment of the child to the mother is neither allowed nor reciprocated by mother (Figure 6-6) in this classic position, which has been termed the one of "evolutionary adaptation" in the human species.

6. In a scene at three months, the child is crying. The mother first observes, then slowly reaches and rocks the cradle briefly. But she does not pick up the baby and offer her body contact. The baby continues to cry.

7. At a picnic at six months, the child is supported in a carrier seat in her mother's lap. She smiles and looks at her mother fondly, and her mother returns the smile and gaze. The baby then arches her back, straining her chest toward her mother. In atypical fashion, the mother remains immobile, with no trace of response in her body (Figure 6-7). The scene ends with the *baby extending her hand* and resting it against her mother's blouse and breast.

8. At nine months, with the child not yet able to support her body in walking, there are several sequences during which the mother and paternal grandmother hold her hands from behind as she takes steps. The girl's pleasure gives way to fatigue and panic which the mother cannot see from behind. She strains up with one arm to try to catch hold of her mother's body and tries to look at her mother. The girl's expression is desperate, yet she is unable to achieve security because her mother keeps walking her forward (Figure 6-8).

9. On a trip to the zoo at fourteen months, the grandmother is holding the child while the mother stands next to them. The child starts a game of taking off her cap and throwing it at her mother, who catches it and replaces in on the child's head. This is repeated over and over. Though both child and mother are smiling, there is a tense and driven quality to the interaction that causes the mother repeatedly to come close to the girl and then step away.

10. Irritability is pronounced at eighteen months. While sitting on the floor, Amy begins to cry. Mother lifts her and promptly places her

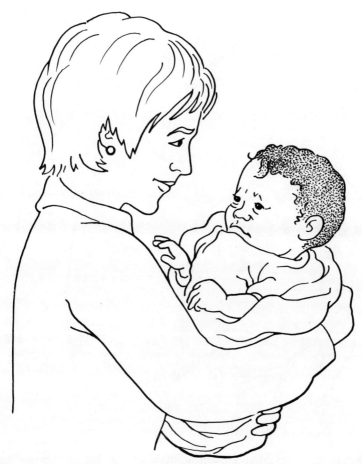

Figure 6.6   2 months. In ventral-ventral position, baby attempts to cling to mother's blouse. But mother does not maintain chest-chest contact or nuzzle baby. The child falls away, unsupported at mother's chest, her irritability heightened.

on the couch without holding her and sits down a few feet away. When the child continues to cry, the mother places her on her knees, facing her but two feet away—without comforting body closeness (Figure 6-9). After a moment, the child throws herself against her mother's chest and the mother's arm limply encircles the child's shoulders. After a few moments, when the child has quieted, the mother plays a game of rocking her forward and back in wide arcs

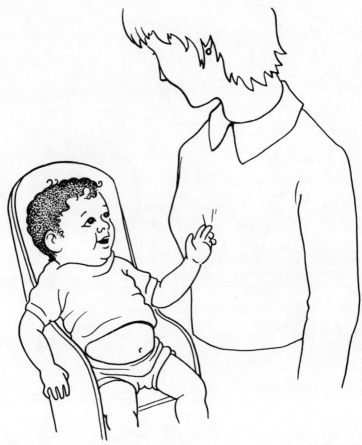

Figure 6.7   6 months. Supported in an infant seat, the baby arches her chest toward mother, smiles broadly at mother's face, and places hand on mother's blouse. Mother returns smile but her torso remains inflexible.

while she is still seated on her knees. Immediately after this, the girl takes a nearby glass and plays a game of pretend drinking, bringing it back and forth from the table to her mouth in wide arcs that recreate the motion and rhythm of the mother's rocking the child moments earlier.

11. In a further scene at eighteen months, Amy is eating and tries to pick up her bottle from the table. However, her hands and the bottle are slippery with food and the bottle keeps slipping from her grasp. She becomes angry and unhappy. Finally the mother inter-

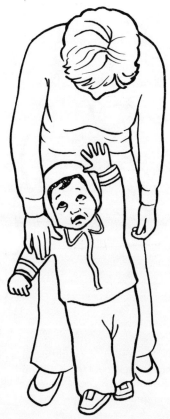

Figure 6.8  9 months. Mother walks child forward by standing behind child and holding her hands from above. Unable to support her weight, the baby panics and reaches desperately for mother's body and tries to see her face. Unaware, mother keeps walking the child forward.

venes, but she only wipes off the bottle. She doesn't help to hold the bottle, or hold it herself, or wipe off the child's hands which are still slippery. As the child continues unsuccessfully to try to pick up the bottle, her tension and anger build until she pounds the table. The scene ends on a Chaplinesque note, with the mother throwing a dishcloth on the table. In a tragicomic manner, the child has struggled against the insurmountable odds of managing her own meal. Finally, she is given her reward—if reward it can be called—a wet dishcloth.

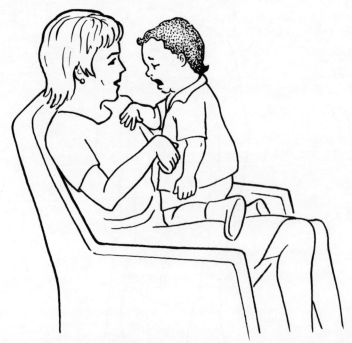

Figure 6.9   18 months. Distressed, the child is placed on the mother's knees, but not brought into chest-chest contact. The child's distress heightens until she throws herself against mother's chest. Note the symmetry of the mother's and child's right hand angulation and gesture.

## INITIAL SIGNS OF ILLNESS

The child's generally somber mood in her first three months may be a prodromal sign. Between twelve and fifteen months, her affect again became somber, and tearfullness, fretfullness, and easy frustration appeared frequently. After fifteen months, there was increasing anger, but affect and expression became generally constricted and wan, with rare slight, brief smiles. At three years, the child's expression was immature, that is, shallow and flat. There was no sense of displeasure or pleasure for more than a moment. There was little involvement in or attentiveness to activities. Affect was little used for communication; rather, it could be called "plastic" because of its easy mutability.

The next seven cases are presented in less detail, in terms of parental background information and discussion of the psychodynamics of the children's conflicts. These briefer cases are nonetheless rich in description, and they emphasize a phenomenological account of the developing signs and symptoms of illness in the children.

### CASE 4 / Edward: Symbiotic Psychosis of Childhood

#### CLINICAL PICTURE

Edward, a male and the youngest of three children, was first suspected to be ill when he was three because of the sudden onset of extreme hyperactivity, negativism, and temper tantrums. His speech began to deteriorate, and gestures took the place of personal pronouns. Prior medical history was negative. Therapists' notes suggested that the mother was controlling of and intrusive into the child's behavior. The boy himself experienced severe separation anxiety when he began nursery school. For weeks he was reduced to helpless rages and wouldn't allow his mother to leave. The father was meek and apologetic with the mother and unable to intervene between mother and child, but he was more realistic in his perceptions of the child. A therapeutic nursery school was begun at four, and intensive outpatient therapy at five, with a diagnosis of symbiotic psychosis of childhood. The case record indicates that after a year of treatment, just as the child was beginning to progress, the mother withdrew him from treatment. Subsequently, he has been in various inpatient and outpatient programs. Now a teenager, he is in a day program. Diagnosed as schizophrenic, he actively hallucinates, is delusional, plays only in parallel with peers, and speaks little and primitively.

#### FILM ANALYSIS

Films began at four months. Analysis revealed that the child's development was unremarkable in the first year. Attachment indicators of molding, lively smiling, looking, and clinging were intact. This was a physically vigorous but somewhat affectively impassive baby. The mother was exceedingly brusque and did not mold to her child. She was rhythmically too brisk for the baby, repeatedly breaking eye contact by turning away from the child to other activities or turning him away. The child's attempts to attach via clinging and eye contact were not reciprocated. In the second year, episodes of rough, perfunctory treatment of the boy by the mother were apparent. In contrast, the father was gentle, synchronized with the child, and showed good molding. At twenty-one months occurs the following sequence which

**TABLE 6-3** *Summary of film observation in Case 3 (Amy). The observations comprise a chronological picture of the mother-infant interaction, child's earliest signs of illness, and child's physical development*

| Age in Months | 0–3 | 3–6 | 6–9 | 9–12 | 12–15 | 15–18 | 18–21 |
|---|---|---|---|---|---|---|---|
| Dyadic gaze between mother and infant | In numerous scenes throughout the first two years, M. and C. initiate, respond, and maintain mutual gazing. | | | | | | |
| Mood of infant and mother | C. is generally somber. | C. shows appropriate distress and irritability when not comforted by M., as well as strong smile in response to M.'s smile. | | | C. is largely somber and fretful. | C. shows increasing anger, but affect generally constricted and wan. | |
| | M. appears largely uncertain, perplexed, and anxious throughout the first two years. | | | | | | |
| Initiation of activity and responsiveness of mother and infant | Scenes in first three months show pattern of M. - C. interaction which characterizes the dyad throughout first years: M.'s chest is wooden. She does not mold to or cuddle child during holding. C. arches toward M., clings, and when distressed presses herself to M.'s chest. | | | | | | |

| | | | |
|---|---|---|---|
| Signs and symptoms of childhood psychosis | | Onset of mood disturbance characterized by somberness and fretfulness. | Mood disturbance broadens with anger and generally constricted, wan affect. |
| Atypical or delayed development | Less than normal activity and attentiveness. Flaccid body tone. More somnolent than normal. | | |

NOTE: Table 6-3 data from film analysis of Case 3. Age of child in months shown horizontally. General categories of observation shown vertically in left column.
C. refers to child. M. refers to mother.

embodied the pattern of earlier interactions. Both parents are in a swimming pool. The mother brusquely pulls the child off the edge of the pool. The father then makes eye contact with the child and holds out his hands to the child who responds by coming to the father. The mother interrupts and competes with the father for the child, taking the boy from the father while the child grimaces and tries to look at his father. The mother returns the child to the father, and the child relaxes.

### INITIAL SIGNS OF ILLNESS

When the films ended at two years, initial signs of illness may have been the increasing impassivity, irritability, and gloomy affect from the second half of the first year of life on.

## CASE 5 / Robert: Autism

### CLINICAL PICTURE

Robert is a male child, the first-born of an identical twinship, and the first born into the family. At fifteen months, the parents became concerned over what appeared to be their child's lack of coordination and took him to an orthopedist. Thence began an odyssey of referrals and treatment programs that seems to have ended when the boy was in his late teens and a resident in a state home for retarded children. Initially there was no finding of orthopedic difficulty, and the child was referred to a pediatrician, who, in turn, referred the case to a child-guidance clinic. No record is available of this evaluation. From ages five to eleven, because of suspected mild cerebral palsy, the child was given an extensive perceptual motor-training program, including rigorous gross and fine motor exercises. At eleven, he was diagnosed as autistic. The parents report that childhood IQ tests were normal and that various medications have not helped.

Behavioral symptoms in early childhood were periods of severe hyperactivity, a toe-walking mannerism, explosive terrors if anything in his environment changed, and lack of relatedness to parents and others. In the parents' words, "As he developed, he never came to anyone to relate any experience or make comments about himself as did his brother . . . he used phrases and then would never use them again." Medical history of gestation revealed a threatened miscarriage at five months and mild toxemia. Developmentally, Robert reached all his motor milestones approximately a month after his brother, but within normal limits. From birth he was smaller than his brother, who has no reported psychiatric illness. The only discrete physical finding has been intermittent bilateral strabismus. No psychiatric evaluation of the parents is available.

## FILM ANALYSIS

Films began at two-and-a-half months and continued to the age of twelve years. In addition to scenes of Robert, there were often scenes of the twin brother, allowing comparison of their development, behavior, and interactions with the parents. Both babies appeared more flaccid and less vigorous than normal controls. Robert was more deviant in this respect. In the first half year, Robert lacked eye pursuit and exploration of his environment; his brother appeared normal. In the first year, Robert's torso often moved stiffly, and his body and limbs moved in an unusually fragmented manner that did not correspond to any known neurologic sign or pathology. Unlike his brother, Robert did not really smile in his first half year, giving instead many fleeting half smiles. The twin brother's primary mood, like Robert's, was irritability, but the brother in his first year showed a full range of well-formed expressions and a strong smile for his mother. Robert achieved all major motor milestones about a month behind his brother, but within normal limits.

The mother's interaction with both children was characterized by physical brusqueness and coercion, and apparent insensitivity to the children's moods or actions. This was not mitigated by gentler behavior. An example at eight months is a bath scene as follows: the brother puts his hand in his mouth and the mother removes it; brother puts a washcloth in his mouth and the mother yanks it away; the brother attempts to put his mouth on the rim of the bath tub and his mother pulls him away. After each removal, the brother looks dejected, while the mother's expression remains inflexibly serious. As the brother tries to mouth an object, he smiles slightly and just as his mouth makes full contact with the object, he smiles more fully. The smile turns to dejection when he is separated from the object. Another scene at ten months showed the mother's brusque, dysrhythmic quality. Both twins were standing at the crib rail. The mother reached out to smooth Robert's hair but instead accidently hit the child's head strongly causing him to grimace and lose his balance. The mother remained self-involved and oblivious to what had just occurred. In holding the children, both parents were very stiff, treating their children like dolls. Like the mother, the father removed Robert's hand from his mouth when he was nine months old, while he was prematurely trying to teach him to play patty-cake.

## INITIAL SIGNS OF ILLNESS

Symptoms were clearly present in this boy at eight-and-a-half months. Sitting in a high-chair, he moved in a bizarre, hyperactive, discoordinated, fragmented way. In other scenes from this period, the child's floppiness and inactivity would shift suddenly to flailing, purposeless hyperactivity. His face had the plastic mutability and the lack of structure of expression and affect (labile shifts from half smiles to grimaces and squints) which eventually constricted to an immature expression. At nine months, the child had repetitive hand-waving autisms. Also at nine months, while the father held Robert who was slumped in his lap, the mother reached to arrange Robert's hands to play patty-cake. Robert struggled away from his parents, flailing with back arched. The parents seemed inflexible and oblivious; they tried neither to control him further nor to soothe him. Their principal mode seemed to be to arrange rather than respond to their children. In scenes at two years, Robert does attend to Christmas presents, though mechanically and tentatively, more like a one-year-old, with an unmodulated excess of energy. He is related enough to approach his mother tentatively when the mother extends her arm to the child. By contrast, the brother molds to his stiff parents nicely throughout. All told, both brothers seemed to be treated equally brusquely and insensitively by the parents, while it is Robert who develops aberrantly.

### CASE 6 / Ethan: Mixed Form of Early Childhood Psychosis

## CLINICAL PICTURE

Ethan was first-born, the son of parents in their mid-twenties. He was first evaluated psychologically at four because of poor speech development, and began day treatment at five. On initial evaluation, he used isolated words or phrases, only rarely communicatively. He never used "I." There was occasional echolalia. He explored inanimate objects, such as toys, with his mouth, and avoided people, including his parents, except to use them mechanically as need-satisfying extensions of himself. This was nevertheless not the intense avoidance many autistics show. There was also anxious fear of strangers, leading to withdrawal. Sometimes Ethan responded—for instance, he might pick up a suggested toy. In his fourth and fifth years, reading comprehension proceeded normally. During this time, Ethan began quoting television commercials, sometimes to communicate. He was diagnosed as a childhood schizophrenic with autistic features.

Additional history from the parents revealed a full-term pregnancy with rare vomiting and slight bleeding. Delivery was by Caesarean section. At three years, the child had a tonsillectomy and at three-and-a-half, a bilateral myringotomy for serous otitis. Neurological workup was normal. The parents had felt the baby to be often vigorous, often quiet. He was weaned from the bottle at two years. In retrospect the parents believe that there was something wrong ("perhaps avoidance") with their child as far back as age one-and-a-half, and noted that in his second year he insisted on baby foods. Developmental history revealed attention to people and objects at two weeks; pleasure and smiling at his parents at one month; reaching to people at two months; much babbling from two months, and isolated words by one year. Major motor milestones were all slightly accelerated. Toilet-training began at two and was completed by four years. He had temper tantrums when frustrated from two to three years, and much clinging to the mother from two to four.

The parents' histories showed severe ongoing marital strife from Ethan's infancy. Mother and father were both tied to their own parents, and when the mother's family moved a long distance away, she made repeated trips there with her son. During one of these trips, when Ethan was two, the father made a serious suicide attempt. Shortly afterwards, the parents entered individual and conjoint therapy. Following what she felt were significant therapeutic gains, the mother reviewed the family movies of Ethan's infancy. She recalled being overprotective of Ethan, but on viewing herself in the movies she spoke of "not being real then (emotionally or physically) . . . just like a doll." For the first time she began to recall strong postpartum feelings of depression and helplessness. Now eight, Ethan remains in day treatment, making modest gains in relatedness and speech use. Prominent, however, are his fears of undertaking new activities and his confusion about relatedness: when he wants his parents, he may smile and go to them simultaneously saying, "Mommy—Daddy go away."

## FILM ANALYSIS

Movies began at two weeks and continued to twenty-eight months. Developmentally, the baby appeared average throughout his first year-and-a-half, neither flaccid and quiet nor highly active. He smiled strongly at his parents by four weeks, and fine and gross motor development were slightly accelerated as in the history. He was a subdued, attentive child who only rarely showed spontaneous pleasure. In his first three years, he was largely curious, gloomy or sad, and irritable. A film scene at three weeks is typical of several from the first two months. Sitting down, the mother holds the baby supine across her lap, angled to her so that his cheek slightly touches her blouse. Inadequately supported, his head slips away. He returns it himself to his mother's blouse. The mother is rocking and cooing, but her torso is planar and boardlike. She moves her face close to the baby's and he responds, shifting from drowsiness to an alert smile. Neither breaks eye contact for about 10 seconds; then the child looks away. The mother's smile has been tense and only half-formed. Tentatively the mother touches the baby's hands and chin through the blankets but makes no further contact. When the child shifts his head and body toward the mother, she doesn't move her body or hands to reciprocate. In another scene, one of feeding at two weeks, the child lies supine alone in the middle of the parents' bed, while the mother sits on the edge of the bed extending the bottle to him from arm's length. These scenes and later ones in the first two years describe parenting that is appropriate but marked by much constraint and seeming perplexity in the mother. By contrast, the father molded to his child when holding him in a fashion typical of parents in the control movies.

### INITIAL SIGNS OF ILLNESS

This boy's generally somber, irritable mien from birth may be a sign of disturbance. By nine months, he is strikingly self-absorbed, not looking at the camera or at people about him. At eleven months, when the mother rolls him a ball he looks at it but does not respond to his mother. His self-absorption mirrors his mother's manner that had been apparent in the films from the early weeks. Between ten and twelve months, there is the beginning of a labile expression—fleeting alternations of pleasure and displeasure—similar to the plasticity of expression seen in other cases, but less intense. At twelve months the boy is somberly content to be held by his mother, but he doesn't look at her and seems unaware of her. In addition, he appears very sad or depressed. Sensitive to his distance, the mother looks at him quizzically, but does not engage him with her eyes, with her voice, with play, or with body stimulation. By sixteen months, Ethan is actively avoiding his mother's and father's attempts to engage him by eye and by toys. Both parents appear dejected. In their frustration, they use inappropriately grown-up toys as a vehicle for interaction. There are no scenes of slowly paced, simple body and toy play. At twelve and sixteen months, the child is exploring new objects frequently with his mouth.

### CASE 7 / Bert: Mixed Form of Early Childhood Psychosis

#### CLINICAL PICTURE

Bert was the second of two children of European immigrants. Both parents had survived wartime tragedies in which they had lost their parents. They met and married in the United States. Bert's older brother was four when Bert was born. The mother recalls being concerned with Bert's lack of response at six months; the family general practitioner is said to have replied that nothing was wrong. The mother also feels that the infant was very sensitive to noises which frequently made him cry. He was irritable, demanding, very active, and showed little pleasure. Until he was about three-and-a-half years old, his parents recalled that he avoided their attempts to play with him, but as he approached four he became increasingly attached to his mother. Medical history, neurologic workup, and electroencephalogram were normal. Pregnancy was uncomplicated, and because of pelvic dystocia delivery was by Caesarean section, as had been that of the older son. Motor milestones were somewhat slow but still normal. For example, Bert did not walk until sixteen months. At this time the child also developed the first of many compulsive rituals. He feared taking food with his hands and demanded that his mother place his food directly in his mouth. For a time at two, he also feared leaving the house with his parents, and he rocked in his bed and sat in a dark closet for periods of time. In his second year, there was also constipation for which his mother gave suppositories. Toilet training was accomplished by four. Speech was very delayed, words appearing at three-and-a-half and sentences at five.

In his first nursery school, Bert kept very distant from peers and because of this, his teacher initiated a referral for psychiatric therapy at age four. On entry into day treatment, Bert had virtually no eye contact and was negativistic. He was diagnosed as suffering from early childhood psychosis. During his years in day treatment, he progressed from isolation and severe inhibition in physical activities to gradual affectionate interaction with classmates and staff. Nonetheless there continued to be outbursts of rage, regressions to self-preoccupation, and fears. Now a teenager, Bert lives in a group home for disturbed adolescents and receives phenothiazines. He is clumsy, grimaces, and has pressured speech. His thinking is concrete and reflects considerable, almost delusional anxiety about being physically hurt in a dangerous world. At times Bert says, with some insight, that his fears are too intense. Compulsive thinking persists in his preoccupation with wiring diagrams and in his memorization of bus routes. There is little further history pertaining to the parents. A note in the case material indicates the mother's tendency to somaticize anxiety; and there are observations of the father's angry physical and verbal outbursts against Bert, his habit of contradicting and controlling his son, and his rigid denial of his own feelings.

## FILM ANALYSIS

The family provided movies that begin at three months and continue to eleven years. The films showed that in the first year, the right corner of the baby's mouth did not go down in smiling or crying; a paralysis or congenital hypoplasia or absence of the *right depressor anguli oris muscle*.[2] This anomaly was less evident in the second year and ultimately almost inapparent. There was also a slight right ptosis in the first half of the first year; it too became inapparent later. These neuromuscular findings had not been previously noted by parents or physicians. Otherwise, the baby in the first six months had good muscle tone. At three months, he had a full social smile, good head and posture control, and was attentive to his mother.

Other major motor milestones were unremarkable. Analysis of the interaction between mother and child showed a mother who was attentive, responsive, and rhythmically attuned to her child. Of the ten cases reported in this chapter, only this mother and Jean's mother had behavior that was indistinguishable from that of control mothers. In a typical interaction at four months, the mother holds and molds to the baby, who likewise molds to her. They are both looking intently at each other. After a few moments the mother looks away, and the child then immediately turns away. A moment later the mother returns her gaze to the child, who follows suit by looking at the mother. The mother's expression is content and smiling without being stiff. On the father's part, however, there are repeated scenes in which he aggressively teases and rebuffs mother and children. He is seen

---

[2]This finding has been reviewed in the *Yearbook of Pediatrics* (1974) where it is suggested that a congenital absence of the *depressor anguli oris* muscle is a relatively common minor anomaly unrelated to other anomalies or perinatal trauma. On the other hand, when the finding represents muscle paralysis secondary to seventh nerve pathology, it is likely to be the result of perinatal trauma or to be associated with other congenital anomalies, especially cardiovascular ones.

throwing snowballs at the family, taking a ball away from the older brother, unaware of the boy's tears, and pinching rather than kissing his wife. He evinces great stiffness and controlled anger.

### INITIAL SIGNS OF ILLNESS

As early as three months, the baby is wan, showing little pleasure or excitement although social smiling is present. He is vacant and does not fix his eyes on people and things, although he does respond to his brother's excitement when they are together. The unfocused, apathetic look is prominent by nine months. At this time there is also self-stimulating, repetitive rocking, and periods of aimless flailing of the whole body. From eight months, there also appear the plastic, fleeting expressions that do not communicate but change swiftly without apparent cause. At twelve months, Bert's body movements decompose just as his facial expression had; he moves his whole body in an unmodulated way, with jerky, athetotic-like dancing movements (autisms) of his fingers. Nonetheless, the child stays close when held by his parents. By one year, the mother is aware of and pained by the child's lack of emotional responsiveness. The father seems unaware and smiles persistently.

## CASE 8 / Steven: Autism

### CLINICAL PICTURE

Steven is the first-born child of parents in their late twenties. His parents first became concerned about him when he was two-and-a-half because of lack of speech development, periods of frenetic overactivity, unresponsiveness, and a repetitive gesture of waving his hand in front of his eyes. Steven was first evaluated at three-and-a-half, diagnosed as autistic, and begun in a therapeutic nursery school. History at initial evaluation revealed that the mother felt that from early in his first year he was very quiet, did not like to be held, avoided eye gaze, and often seemed unaware of people. These were also salient behaviors at evaluation. From early in the first year, feeding was difficult, the mother being unsure when Steven was hungry, and there was a great deal of gagging and vomiting. The mother could not recollect a responsive smile. She recalled that he played peek-a-boo and patty-cake from about nine months, and had a security blanket. Motor milestones occurred somewhat slowly but within normal limits. Toilet training was completed at four. A striking feature of Steven's history is that at about three years of age he had taught himself to read, a precocity that he has maintained throughout his schooling. Medical history has been negative; results of initial neurologic workup are not available, but there are no present neurologic findings. The mother suffered a flu-like illness in the second trimester of pregnancy and, later, headache and edema. Steven's birth weight was 7½ pounds.

Since his first evaluation at four to his present age of ten, Steven has attended a series of therapeutic schools. In these six years, he has progressed from isolation to gradual affiliation with peers, and from autistic states to group and interpersonal participation with a need for rigidly routinized activities. Temper tantrums and head-banging persist when he is frustrated. Recently Steven has begun to hear voices and talk to them, and has been diagnosed as schizophrenic. His intellectual endowment is very high, and he is gifted in memorization and mathematics. The Project has had no first-hand contact with this family, and reports from evaluating and therapeutic institutions have not included a psychodynamic formulation of the family constellation and of the boy's illness. One educational institution observed, however, the parents' insistence on cleanliness, and correlated this with the child's constriction in play.

## FILM ANALYSIS

The family movies began during pregnancy and continued into the child's seventh year. The mother's sister-in-law delivered her first child a week after Steven was born, and several scenes allowed comparison of the two mothers' behaviors with their infants and of the infants' responsiveness. In the films, Steven's motor development appeared normal; bonding responses to his mother were present in the first three months, and his level of activity was unremarkable. Analysis of social interaction yielded many interesting observations. During pregnancy the mother was observed to be stiff, conscious of her appearance, and involved in grooming herself (and in one scene, her sister-in-law as well); she straightens her sister-in-law's blouse with a quick gesture which neither sister-in-law nor Mrs. O. seem aware of. When the child is born and throughout his first six months, the mother does not mold to him: her thorax is planar rather than segmental in movement, and she fusses with the infant's clothes without holding him close or touching him. Her expression is fixed in a tense, somewhat angry smile. In every respect the sister-in-law appears more relaxed.

For his part, Steven is generally more irritable than his infant cousin. In feeding scenes at three and five months, a battle is apparent. The mother forcefully, if not angrily, pushes the child's head into position to receive the spoon. The baby is angry and does not make eye contact with his mother. By this time, the child has a somber mood and rarely shows pleasure. There are no scenes in which the parents face their child while playing with him. A striking and representative scene occurs at about five months. The mother, seated behind the child and partially supporting him as he sits, bounces a teddy bear in his lap. Just as the boy begins to show pleasure (which seems in response to genital and physical stimulation), the mother leaves. The baby's expression turns to bewilderment, then confusion, then somber wanness. He falls from the sitting position and lies limp and depressed. This sequence is repeated twice, the mother stopping each time a smile begins to form on the baby's face. The mother's rhythm throughout is too rapid for the baby. The rare scenes of father and child mirror the mother's tenseness, lack of reciprocity with the baby, and lack of awareness of the boy's mood or rhythm.

### INITIAL SIGNS OF ILLNESS

These may have been his somberness and avoidance of eye contact as early as three months. At twelve months, there were aimless hand-opening and closing movements, as well as plasticity of expression in this generally grim baby in the form of fleeting near-smiles arising without apparent external stimuli. In the second year, the plasticity continued in aimless, formless, and uncommunicative expressions; Steven became less and less attentive to people, although he did occasionally respond to his parents' instructions, and a hand-flapping stereotypie appeared.

### CASE 9 / Jean: Autism

#### CLINICAL PICTURE

Jean's case was first reported by Erik Erikson in *Childhood and Society* (1950) in the chapter "Early Ego Failure." Erikson provided consultation for Jean and her family when she was between six and ten years. Because her illness was advanced and resisted therapy, at eleven she was transferred to residential treatment. Since then she has had a long series of inpatient and outpatient therapeutic programs, increasingly supportive in nature. In her middle thirties, Jean left her last residential setting and now, in her early forties, she lives with her mother. Many of the childhood behaviors described by Erikson appear now in Jean's middle life like the qualities of a severely eccentric adult. She is often subdued and sometimes impulsive, with some posturing. Although her speech is fragmented and parroting, she sometimes speaks perceptively and empathically. Largely alone, Jean does some housework, walks in the neighborhood, paints, and goes on outings with groups for the handicapped.

In his case history, Erikson describes an extremely traumatic childhood in which Jean suffered from severe thrush in the first six months of life, requiring surgical excision of infected skin at one point. In addition, the mother developed tuberculosis and though treated at home, she was isolated in her bedroom between Jean's seventh and eleventh month. Shortly before being separated from her mother, Jean had lost her kind and gentle nurse who was replaced by a tough, emphatic, disapproving nurse whose favorite remark was, according to the mother, "Ah, baby you stink."

The mother described how, when she was reunited with her baby after four months, the child "shrank back from the pattern of chintz on the armchair and . . . cried all the time." Jean's fears extended to many things, and although her motor development progressed normally, she became sadder, quieter, and avoided closeness with her older brother and parents. Objects such as a sheet and pillows became the recipients of her affection, and she related to people as if they were fragments or parts of whole people with qualities that might damage her or whom she herself might destroy if she stayed too close.

In addition to Erikson's published report, the case records from several institutions were reviewed. They showed that other than the thrush, Jean's childhood was unremarkable medically. The pregnancy was complicated by bleeding in the first trimester. Notes record that the mother was maternal in her concern and actions. She herself recalled being emotionally upset at the birth of the child, and wondered if the tuberculosis might not have been precipitated by emotional factors. The record indicates that there was in fact a series of severe and controlling women caring for Jean, of whom the angry nurse was but one. The father was rigid, dominating, and compulsively fearful of dirt; the mother was submissive to him, as well as to the autocratic women who cared for Jean in her early years.

## FILM ANALYSIS

Movies follow Jean from birth to ten years. Developmentally, in the first week the baby is alert and active with good body tone. Her hands go to her mouth for comfort, and she molds to the chest of the nurse holding her. When the side of her mouth is stimulated, she has strong cardinal points and rooting reflexes. At one month, she is seen initiating and making good eye contact with the nurse bathing her. At two months, in a scene in which she is held in the ventral-ventral position, the baby clings and molds strongly. Also at two months there is a pronounced full smile. Until five months, her affect is an unremarkable mixture of displeasure and pleasure; and throughout her early childhood, Jean's gross and fine motor development appear to progress normally.

Analysis of social interaction yielded but two observations of the mother with the baby in the first year, for the mother was the principal photographer, capturing the child with others. In a scene at about five months, the mother warmly holds Jean to her chest and Jean rests comfortably, smiles, and reaches for her mother's face. At about seven months, while bathing the child, the mother twice removes the child's hands from the child's mouth. Then the baby raises her left hand and stares at it blankly, seemingly not noticing the mother. The mother turns the child's head around somewhat sharply in order to make eye contact with her. In the first week, there are several scenes of the nurse holding Jean. She handles the baby brusquely; she takes Jean's hands out of her mouth and ignores the baby's heightening irritation. In one scene at three days, as the nurse holds the irritable child up for the camera, her left hand inadvertently brushes the right side of the child's mouth (one of the cardinal reflex points). Jean's mouth opens wide and she turns her head toward the nurse's chest; the nurse remains immobile, offering no ventral-ventral contact, and Jean's head falls away, her limbs flailing. At one month, the nurse brusquely and rapidly bathes the baby with no play, eye, or body contact. The baby attempts to make eye contact, but the nurse either knocks or splashes the baby's head, and the baby turns away. Early in the second year, both mother and father appear more frequently in play with their children. At sixteen months, the mother kneels down next to Jean, who is sitting. She brings Jean close to her and looks smilingly at her. Jean returns the gaze rather vacantly. The mother then starts to back away, slowly and relaxedly holding her hands out to Jean. Jean looks at her, takes a few steps toward her, and then turns away. Seen in the second year for the first time, the father is as gentle and patient as the mother in this scene.

## INITIAL SIGNS OF ILLNESS

These include Jean's vacant, unfocused look and her preferring to look at her hand rather than her mother's face at seven months. At eleven months, Jean was seen rocking back and forth with a vacant expression. At twelve months, there is an instance of aimless flailing. By this time, symptoms of illness are striking. Sitting on her mother's lap, her mother smiling at her, Jean seems unaware of her. Jean rocks to and fro, making repetitive up-and-down waving movements (autisms) with her fingers. At her first birthday, she averts her face from eye contact with her mother and father, a mannerism that becomes more prominent as time passes. Her expression does not mature, but increasingly has a lost or quizzical look that shifts in a plastic and uncommunicative manner into fleeting smiles, grimaces, coy glances, and confusion.

### CASE 10 / Ken: Autism

#### CLINICAL PICTURE

Ken was a first-born child of parents in their early twenties. He was first referred for therapy in his third year by the family's pediatrician and by the nursery school teacher. They noticed the child's increasing restlessness, his attention to objects rather than to people or his parents, and his controlling behavior with his mother. At three-and-a-half years, Ken was begun in a day-treatment program and gradually moved into full hospitalization at another institution, which continued for many years to offer milieu and individual therapy for the child and individual and conjoint therapy for the parents. When treatment began, Ken used phrases for communication, but had speech reversals and neologisms and used no personal pronouns. He engaged in long periods of repetitive, tense vertical jumping and dirt sifting; he was rigid in his needs for routine, and often negative and aggressive; he also showed little difficulty in separating from his parents. A quality of distraction in the boy led staff to suspect that he was hallucinating. Medical and neurologic workups were negative. He was initially diagnosed as autistic but available for interaction, and as time passed, the diagnosis was changed to childhood schizophrenia.

Contact with the parents made the staff aware of how unusual they were. The mother kept up a steady stream of talk with staff and her husband. She was severely controlling of both her husband's and her son's behavior. Though profoundly concerned about her son, she expressed ambivalence, if not hostility, in her comments about him. For example, she often overwhelmed him with effusive hugging, while at the same time she might say, "You're such a good boy I could eat you up." The child physically withdrew from her too rapid and forceful attention. Overt aggression broke through when she some-times struck Ken. The father had a strong need for Ken to demonstrate any accomplishment to the staff. Consequently he was generally insensitive and inappropriate in his attempts to force his son to perform. The parents' therapy later uncovered their long-standing insecurity and fear of criticism, intense to the point of clinical paranoia. The mother related that she had felt inferior to her own mother from early in Ken's life. She recalled that in childhood she had been impulsive, eccentric, and had little social contact with classmates. She was obsessively concerned about keeping everything in its place at home. In her son's early childhood, she was distressed about the illness of her sister who died when Ken was three. The father was largely raised by surrogate parents while his natural parents were involved in business activities.

Ken's gestation and neonatorium were normal, and developmental milestones occurred at the expected times. At four months, however, the child was rapidly weaned and placed on a rigid feeding schedule so that the mother could leave him for a week's vacation. At about this time, the parents feel their son began to avert his gaze from them and rock in his crib with hands clenched. Because he would cry when his mother removed him from the play pen, he was increasingly left there alone. Bowel training took place from nine to fifteen months. Between sixteen and twenty-four months, he had a series of severe and painful ear infections associated with head banging. During this period the mother feels the child looked at her with hatred. Ken's therapeutic progress was slow, but after ten years of both day and residential treatment with two successive therapists, he was returned to his parents' home and is now in an ordinary high school. Parents and child continue in supportive therapy, and Ken is felt now to be still obsessive-compulsive, but not psychotic.

In view of some of the film data to follow, a segment of his therapeutic process is of interest. It comes from the period about a year before discharge (age twelve), when Ken was able to verbalize feelings, and it reflects his fears of being controlled, his anger, and his need for closeness. Ken and the therapist are wrestling:

> Ken: "I'd like to mangle you [the therapist] and cut you up in little pieces."
> Therapist: "You're angry."
> Ken: "No, I'm always happy."
> Therapist: "Most people are sad at times."

> Ken: "I know how I feel and it's better to be happy."
> Therapist: "I get sad and even cry at times."
> Ken: "I'm not going to be sad when I leave [the hospital]; you're going to be sad old man . . . let's wrestle."
>
> After a few moments Ken adds:
>
> Ken: "I like wrestling better than you holding me for throwing things on the floor. . . . I need holding sometimes to get relaxed. . . ."

## FILM ANALYSIS

The movies began at one month and continued to seven years. There were no neurologic findings; this baby appeared vigorous and alert. There were numerous scenes in the first three months in which the child reached toward and grasped his mother's torso and rested his hand on her breast when close. Attentive, he gazed at his parents and others' movements about him.

Social-interaction analysis of child and the parents yielded much more malignant findings. Both mother and father were seen frequently and were remarkably similar in behavior. From the first scenes at one month, the mother was awkward. Holding the child, her arms were stiff, a quality that only slightly eased as time passed. At one-and-a-half months, the mother looked uncomfortable playing with the baby. She overstimulated him and controlled all maintenance and termination of activity between them. When the infant made eye contact with her, she looked at him and quickly turned him away to the camera. Here, and at other times, there is no reciprocal play between parent and child. The baby is, however, given autonomy in mouthing his pacifier. In a scene at six months that is repeated at other times, the mother brings the child into close chest-chest contact with her. She then frenetically stimulates the boy by jiggling, rocking, and swaying him with no pause to observe or share in the child's response to these activities. The father too is compulsively active with his son, often roughly turning him out to the camera and pushing him to perform a task, unaware of the child's mood. For example, at twenty-eight months, the father places the boy on a rocking horse and rapidly pushes him up and down. The child's expression shifts between fragmented smiles and distress. Finally the child gets off the horse, lets himself fall to the floor, then slowly rolls over on his stomach, expressionless. In an earlier scene at about eighteen months, the mother's overstimulation (as well as inferable hostility) took the form of her bouncing a ball off the child's head in play.

## INITIAL SIGNS OF ILLNESS

Signs appeared between three and six months when Ken was increasingly self-engaged with his rattle and his teething toy while his mother was active with him. At six months, he seemed oblivious and content to focus on a pacifier when his mother bodily moved him about. At eighteen months, he was engaged in intense autoerotic bouncing, and his body was becoming unusually rigid. His affect by this time was largely a constricted partial smile that often broke down into distress. By three years, he had a stereotypic sway to his walk at times, and held his arms in a rigid, disjointed manner. He made little response to other children. Nonetheless, throughout childhood there were instances when the boy continued to make affective contact with and respond to his parents.

# Conclusion

These case histories suggest correlations between the innate characteristics of the children, styles of parenting, environmental factors, and the psychotic symptomatology of the children. In addition, the studies demonstrate connections between overt behavior and the internal psychological states of the parents and infants. However, the first intent of this chapter has been to bring to life the earliest months of these children's and parents' lives together in a narrative-like form, deriving data from various sources. From this we can cull recurring observations and draw psychodynamically oriented inferences about the ten case studies.

The anguish of parents who become aware of the unresponsiveness of their children repeatedly confronts us. So does the distress of infants who were pushed away, not looked at, or not allowed to engage in a reciprocity with their parents that involves the modalities of bonding, emotional confirmation, and affectionate interchange. As we said earlier, the reciprocity of the parent-child relationship, especially that of the mother and baby, teaches the infant reliable methods of tension reduction, and maintains an internal and interpersonal equilibrium before tension builds to disorganizing levels. In this process, the ego becomes structuralized as it begins the intrapsychic process of self-other differentiation and the gradual development of autonomous ego functioning. While the major hypotheses that can be derived from the Early Natural History of Childhood Psychosis Project appear in Chapter 10, several of the cases draw attention to striking patterns of the mother-infant interaction that appear in

**TABLE 6-4** *Atypical signs in the infancy home movies of ten cases of early childhood psychosis*

| | Signs of Atypical Development | 1 | 2 | 3 | 4 | 5 | 6 | 7 | 8 | 9 | 10 |
|---|---|---|---|---|---|---|---|---|---|---|---|
| | | | | | | | | Case Number | | | |
| Birth to 6 months | Flaccid body tone | 1 | 3 | 2 | | 3 | | | | | |
| | Lacks attentiveness or response to people or things | 2 | 3 | | 4 | 3 | 9 | 3 | 12 | 6 | |
| | Lacks excitement in presence of parents | 4 | 3 | | | | 9 | | 24 | 6 | |
| | Lacks anticipatory posturing to being picked up | | 3 | | | | | | | | |
| | Vacant, unfocused gaze | 9 | | | | | 16 | 3 | 24 | 6 | 5 |
| | Less than normal activity (e.g., reaching) | 2 | 3 | 2 | | 3 | | | | | |
| | Specific motor deviations: a. Developmental head lag on being pulled to sitting | | 6 | | | | | | | | |
| | b. Submental palsy | | | | | | | 3 | | | |
| | c. Ptosis | | | | | | | 3 | | | |
| | Doesn't mold to mother's body | | 5 | | | | | | | | |
| | Eye-squint mannerism | | 3 | | | | | | | | |
| | Predominantly somber or irritable mood; little smiling | 9 | 5 | 3 | 12 | 3 | 1 | 8 | 3 | | |
| | More somnolent than normal | | 3 | 2 | 4 | | | | | | |
| 6–12 months | Seeming hallucinatory excitement | 9 | | | | | | | | | |
| | Appears self-absorbed | 7 | 7 | | | | 9 | | 24 | 6 | 7 |
| | No visual pursuit of people | 6 | 7 | | | 3 | 9 | | | | |
| | Looks away from people repeatedly | | 7 | | | | | | | | 12 |
| | Avoids mother's gaze | 6 | 7 | | | | 16 | | | | 12 |

**TABLE 6-4** *(Continued)*

| | Signs of Atypical Development | 1 | 2 | 3 | 4 | 5 | 6 | 7 | 8 | 9 | 10 |
|---|---|---|---|---|---|---|---|---|---|---|---|
| | | | | | | Case Number | | | | | |
| 6–12 months | Resists being held; arches torso away from parents on being held | | 5 | | | 9 | | | | | |
| 6–12 months | Autisms: a. Hand flapping | 9 | 12 | | | 9 | | 12 | 12 | | 12 |
| 6–12 months | b. Finger-dancing movements | 9 | | | | | | 12 | | | 12 |
| 6–12 months | c. Rocking | | | | | | | 9 | | | 11 |
| 6–12 months | Plastic expressions—fleeting, unstructured, not communicating affect or intention; labile shifts from grimaces to squints | 12 | | | | 9 | 10 | 8 | 12 | 18 | 12 |
| 6–12 months | Fragmented, uncoordinated body movements | | | | | 9 | | 12 | | 18 | 12 |
| 6–12 months | Episodes of flailing, aimless, unmodulated hyperactivity | | | | | 9 | | 9 | | 18 | 12 |
| 12–24 months | Doesn't approach parents | 9 | | | | | 16 | | | | |
| 12–24 months | Keeps distance from parents | 9 | 12 | | | | | | | | |
| 12–24 months | Constricted or flattened affect | 9 | 7 | 15 | | | 16 | | 24 | 18 | |
| 12–24 months | Little or no purposeful activity | 15 | | | | 24 | | | | 18 | 12 |

NOTE: Signs of atypical development in first two years seen in ten cases later diagnosed as early childhood psychosis. Left-hand column indicates findings in period of life that they were frequently first observed. Right-hand columns indicate the month of life that each finding was first seen in a given case. (Ages are sometimes approximate since subject to clinical judgment.)

the earliest months of the lives of subsequently ill children. These important configurations may be characterized as follows:

*Pattern 1: A mother paradoxically stimulating of and avoidant of eye gaze with her baby, and an initially responsive child.* This is exemplified by Case 1 where a major modality of bonding—mutual eye gaze—received interference by the mother in a manner that could be termed a *preverbal double bind.* Rather than verbalizing conflicting instructions and feelings to her infant as may occur later in families when children understand and speak (Bateson et al., 1956), the mother affectionately physically stimulated her child; yet seconds later her ambivalence toward the baby undercut her affection, and she withdrew from the baby's attempts to meet her gaze. The infant, observably confused and dejected in scenes at four months, became progressively withdrawn in the second six months until clear autistic symptoms were present by the end of the first year.

*Pattern 2: An unresponsive infant and a wooden, ungiving mother.* Exemplified by Case 2, the pronounced characteristic in this dyad is the mother's lack of activity across the range of bonding modalities— her stiffness and slowness of response which was not enlivened by warmth and excitement. However, there were no traumatic distortions or omissions of response. The infant, too, was without life. Symptoms of childhood psychosis emerged in the second six months of life.

*Pattern 3: A mother unable to allow bonding and reduce her child's tension through patient and close gentle holding, and a responsive infant.* Because of her own perplexity, self-doubts, and lack of external affectionate support, the mother in Case 3 was unable to perceive and respond to rising states of distress in her baby by holding her close. The infant, on her part, was responsive; however, as the initial responsivity was not reciprocated by the mother, she became increasingly clinging, demanding, and unable to develop age-appropriate toddler autonomy. Case 10 resembled this, but in addition, the parents were extremely physically over-stimulating of their child, which further interfered with bonding.

*Pattern 4: Adequate parenting and an unresponsive infant.* In Case 7, the mother was warm, responsive, and indistinguishable from the most nurturing of control-group mothers. However her baby— stigmatized by minor neurologic findings of congenital or perinatal origin—remained apathetic and withdrawn. Between nine and twelve months of age, clear symptoms of early childhood psychosis appeared.

These patterns of disturbed mother-infant functioning were teased out from the rich case material presented above. They do not demonstrate a simple cause-effect relationship between the parent-infant disturbances and childhood psychosis; instead, they are a descriptive rendering of some subtle, and some more obvious forms of pathological interaction and psychic states. Their determinants and permutations may be uncovered in many areas of the families' emotional lives and activities. Other families with disturbance present still further variations of these patterns. Finally, what is most striking in these cases is the unfolding of the pathognomonic symptoms of childhood psychosis from the earliest mother-child relationship and family interaction.

Table 6-4 summarizes the unfolding of signs of atypical development in the ten children reported in this chapter. The left-hand column lists these findings. The top section of the left-hand column groups those signs that were most frequently observed in the children from birth to six months. The right-hand columns show the month of life that a finding first appeared on the films of a child. For example, Case 1 demonstrated *a lack of attentiveness or response to people or things* at two months, and Case 2 at three months. By contrast, this sign appeared in Case 6 at nine months and Case 8 at twelve months; but the table still groups this sign during the birth-to-six-months period since it appeared most frequently at this time in most of the other cases. The signs of the first six months are prodromal to illness. They are also nonspecific developmental deviations that may be shown by many normal children who continue their growth without any illness or further maturational disturbance.

However, another cluster of signs appeared in most cases between six and twelve months, and these are so grouped in Table 6-4. For example, Cases 1 and 5 evidenced *hand flapping* at nine months; Cases 2, 7, 8 and 10, at twelve months. The signs of this period indicate clearly developing pathology in the children if they persist and are not just transient manifestations. Between twelve and twenty-four months, Table 6-4 lists a third clustering of findings. These are *symptoms* in a child of established early childhood psychosis—*not approaching the parents, keeping a distance from the parents, constricted or flattened affect,* and *little or no purposeful activity.* It is striking that nine of the ten children had clear pathology by twelve months of age, as evidenced by somber moods, avoidance of parental gaze, resistance to being held, stereotypic mannerisms, plastic, labile, and flattened expressions, and distancing from parents. Of these same nine children, there was no professional recognition of illness and commencement of treatment until months, and most often years later, when the pathologic process was already firmly established and the prognosis for improvement grim.

# Chapter 7

## Blind Ratings of Mother-Infant Interaction in Home Movies of Prepsychotic and Normal Infants

In early phases of the Early Natural History of Childhood Psychosis Project, the methodology was a systematized form of clinical observation. Cases were selected for study in which the investigators were already familiar with the psychopathological outcome of the children. And as stated in Chapter 6, the most significant findings that emerged from close examination of the premorbid infancy films were: (1) the absence of symptoms of psychosis in the first six months of life; (2) the appearance of distinct symptoms in most children at about twelve months, with the delineation of the subjects' failure to gain at this time the age-appropriate ability to communicate affect, meaning, and intention through facial expression; and (3) apparent failures of/or dampened responsiveness of parent to baby and vice versa in many families, beginning as early as the first weeks of life. In the process of identifying these aberrancies, we also recognized five key modalities of mother and infant behavior that were related to reciprocal interaction in the first six months of life—eye gaze, touching, holding, affect, and feeding. Vocalization was also present but not studied because the movies did not have sound.

The findings were of heuristic value, but because the investigators were familiar with the children's diagnoses, they could not validate etiologic hypotheses which related aberrancies in the early mother-infant interaction to childhood psychosis. The next step in the research, therefore, was to determine if there was statistical significance to the subjective clinical impressions, and to test more rigorously the hypotheses generated in the clinical studies. This was done by obtaining a control group of home movies and having judges, blind to the developmental outcome of the child and to the hypotheses of the study, give ratings to several parameters which had been recognized as constituting the mother-infant interaction.

There were two major foci of this endeavor, based on the outcome of the clinical analysis. First, because of the finding that symptoms of the childhood psychosis did not appear in the first six months of life, we wanted to test whether there were differences in bonding and attachment behaviors between the index and control-group families during this period. This could potentially point to predictors of childhood psychosis in the earliest months of the infants' lives that would be based on observable behaviors in the mother-infant interaction. The theoretical rationale for this grows from the studies reviewed in Chapters 3 and 4 which make clear that the infant indeed has some sophistication in communicating affective and physiologic states and needs, and that the earliest mother-child behavior builds on the infant's communicative capacities in a way that is significant for development.

The second focus of testing in this substudy was to document aberrant mother-infant dyadic avoidance and reciprocity in the subsequently psychotic children. Case studies of the Project in Chapter 6 had suggested that very early patterns of mother-infant dyadic avoidance and reciprocity appeared to be longitudinally incorporated into and to characterize the child's later symptomatology. From the case studies, we expected that there would be more reciprocal interactive behavior between the control infants and their mothers and less withdrawal from this than in the index group. While there is no manifest psychotic symptomatology in the index infants in the first six months of life, whether differences occurred in the maternal behaviors, in the infant behaviors, and in the quality of the mother-infant interaction between the control and index groups needed to be tested.

The hypotheses for testing were as follows:

1. In the first six months of life, we would expect higher scores for mothers and infants in the control group in the variables of eye gaze, holding, touching, affect, and feeding than in the index group;
2. We would expect greater reciprocity and less avoidance in the control group than the index group.

## Data Base

While the index-case movies were largely obtained through treatment institutions and announcements in parent-group newsletters requesting home movies to study the early life of subsequently ill children, the controls were obtained through announcements in nonpsychiatric institutional media for home movies for the study of child development. The movies of four index cases in addition to those discussed in Chapter 6 were obtained for this phase of the Project. The overall sample consisted of the home movies of fourteen subsequently psychotic children and fourteen controls. The samples were matched for numbers of first- and second-born. Demographically and ethnically, the groups were well-matched. All of the families were at least second generation residents of the United States, except for one immigrant family in each group. The index group was skewed toward a slightly lower socioeconomic status than the control families. There was no indication of defective intelligence or nutritional deprivation in any families of the two groups. At least one parent was employed in all of the families. Table 7-1 summarizes the characteristics of the research population.

## Methodology

Two types of ratings were done: individual ratings of both mothers and infants on the five bonding/attachment variables listed above, and global assessments of attachment.

Because the raw data base was naturalistic and nonstandardized, the methodology had to be adapted to this unusual data. To do this, we established strict criteria (1) of consistency in choosing segments of film for rating, and (2) of reliability in interrater agreement among the judges making the ratings. We used the following procedure.

TABLE 7-1    *Characteristics of the sample*

|  | Index group (N = 14) | Control group (N = 14) |
|---|---|---|
| Sex of child |  |  |
| Boys | 11 | 9 |
| Girls | 3 | 5 |
| Birth order of child |  |  |
| First-born boys | 9 | 7 |
| Later-born boys | 2 | 2 |
| First-born girls | 2 | 4 |
| Later-born girls | 1 | 1 |
| Ethnicity |  |  |
| Causasian | 12 | 13 |
| Non-caucasian | 2 | 1 |
| S.E.S. |  |  |
| Professional | 7 | 10 |
| White collar | 5 | 3 |
| Blue collar | 2 | 1 |
| Mother's age |  |  |
| 35 years or older | 3 | 0 |
| Less than 35 years | 11 | 14 |

### Selection of Film Segments

There was a different number of ratable segments for each subject. To provide standardization so that each rater was observing and rating the same segment, one of the investigators and an assistant viewed all of the film footage for each control and index child to ascertain the demarcation point between the events of the first six months of the subjects' lives and later film events. The reliability between the two viewers (percentage of agreement out of total choices) in determining this six-month cut-off point was 0.92. The age of the child was determined by the methodology previously outlined in Chapter 5 (and repeated in Chapter 8).

Then to attain maximum information from our data and also to achieve as much standardization of the data as possible, we chose an equal number of ratable segments for each attachment/bonding parameter for both index and control groups. The criteria for the selection of segments to rate, and the attachment/bonding parameters therein, were these. We chose segments which best captured the variable under consideration by dint of the clarity of the behavior as a function of its duration on film, the quality of the film, and the visability of the particular interaction as a result of the camera angle. In other words, the segments of film had to be adequate to capture the behavior that was to be given a rating. No more than one attachment/bonding variable was rated per segment. The variable being rated had to be in the context of the mother-child interaction. For example, if a mother was with the father, but without her infant, it would be possible to observe her affect; however, we did not rate such instances.

Once segments had been selected for rating on the basis of clarity of mother-infant interaction, the researcher and assistant then independently chose the particular attachment/bonding parameter for scoring. That is, they independently decided which variable was best presented on film for rating in a given segment. In this they agreed 85 percent of the time. The segments and variable selected were marked for the blind observers. Although the total amount of film footage for each subject was quite varied (see Table 8-1, column 2) for the first six months of the subjects' lives, we had relatively comparable amounts of footage across index and control cases. When the total frequency of ratable segments was calculated and marked for the raters, there were four ratable segments for holding, touching, eye gaze, and affect for each control and index case. There were three ratable segments of feeding for eleven of the control cases and eight of the index cases. For three of the control cases and six of the index cases, there were two ratable feeding segments.

When the film preparers could not agree on the particular attachment/bonding parameter for rating, it was because mothers and infants in reality may show more than one bonding and attachment behavior at a given interactional moment. We chose to rate one behavior for each section of film footage for the mother and child. This choice was to avoid a halo effect that might arise, for example, if we observed an interaction in which both touching and holding variables were observed with sufficient clarity to assign a rating; if the first variable, touching, received a high rating, this score might influence the rating of holding in a higher direction than it deserved. To avoid such a halo effect in instances where there was more than one ratable attachment/bonding variable, we used randomized statistical techniques to select the segment for observation. There were three instances in which such a problem arose, and these were related to eye gaze and affect. The reliabilities later achieved by the blind judges scoring these randomized segments were as high as those for the nonrandomized segments.

## The Rating Scale

The Project then developed a 5-point scale to rate the five variables of eye gaze, touching, holding, affect, and feeding. Termed the Early Natural History of Childhood Psychosis Project Scale of Mother-Infant Attachment Indicators (see Appendix), the instrument assessed the intensity of the mothers' or infants' attachment to the other. This scale goes from a low value of 1 (indicative of maternal or infant aversion and isolation) to a high value of 5 (indicative of intense anxious responsiveness and clinging). Both 1 and 5 represent pathologic extremes and 3 represents normative behavior. However, for statistically computing the blind ratings, the scaling was adjusted to be interval-like by having 1 represent the least optimal rating and 5 the most optimal response for a given attachment/bonding behavior. The three raters for the study, who were undergraduate psychology majors, received instruction in the use of the scale over a period of several weeks. The training employed standardized films of mother-infant interactions before, during, and after a feeding. This allowed study not only of the feeding, but also of the range of bonding variables upon which the project focused. The training also used one of the home movies to accustom the raters to the rating of the actual data. Two sets of interrater reliabilities were obtained, using Pearson Product Moment Correlations. The first followed the instruction period and indexed the rater's abilities to apply the scales, in this case to ten training films. Table 7-2 lists the reliabilities achieved both on practice films and subsequently on the index and control movies.

## Procedure for Rating

The procedure for rating the segments of the home movies was as follows. The control and index movies were assigned to the raters in random order. Each rater looked at the films independently, with the scenes and attachment/bonding behavior for rating designated, which allowed him to go back and observe a scene as many times as necessary to make an adequate judgment as to the specific bonding behaviors that best described a particular scene. Kodak M95 Dual 8 mm projectors were used with single-frame and slow-motion capacity.

Then the raters assigned global ratings of attachment for the

**TABLE 7-2  Interrater reliabilities for training and ratings of study**

*Training reliabilities: Interrater reliabilities for variables from 10 training films*

|  | Infant eye gazing | Infant touch | Infant holding | Infant affect | Infant feeding |
|---|---|---|---|---|---|
| Rater 1–Rater 2 | .75 | .81 | .83 | .69 | .75 |
| Rater 1–Rater 3 | .79 | .80 | .84 | .61 | .74 |
| Rater 2–Rater 3 | .70 | .75 | .79 | .65 | .73 |
|  | $\bar{x} = .75$ | $\bar{x} = .79$ | $\bar{x} = .82$ | $\bar{x} = .65$ | $\bar{x} = .74$ |

|  | Mother eye gazing | Mother touch | Mother holding | Mother affect | Mother feeding |
|---|---|---|---|---|---|
| Rater 1–Rater 2 | .82 | .87 | .79 | .70 | .85 |
| Rater 1–Rater 3 | .85 | .85 | .75 | .62 | .79 |
| Rater 2–Rater 3 | .79 | .85 | .85 | .68 | .84 |
|  | $\bar{x} = .82$ | $\bar{x} = .86$ | $\bar{x} = .80$ | $\bar{x} = .67$ | $\bar{x} = .83$ |

*Study reliabilities: Interrater reliabilities for blind ratings of home movies*

|  | Infant eye gazing | Infant touch | Infant holding | Infant affect | Infant feeding |
|---|---|---|---|---|---|
| Rater 1–Rater 2 | .78 | .75 | .67 | .65 | .85 |
| Rater 1–Rater 3 | .75 | .69 | .75 | .59 | .88 |
| Rater 2–Rater 3 | .81 | .70 | .69 | .64 | .86 |
|  | $\bar{x} = .78$ | $\bar{x} = .71$ | $\bar{x} = .70$ | $\bar{x} = .63$ | $\bar{x} = .86$ |

|  | Mother eye gazing | Mother touch | Mother holding | Mother affect | Mother feeding |
|---|---|---|---|---|---|
| Rater 1–Rater 2 | .80 | .79 | .72 | .78 | .89 |
| Rater 1–Rater 3 | .76 | .85 | .75 | .75 | .91 |
| Rater 2–Rater 3 | .77 | .69 | .74 | .76 | .90 |
|  | $\bar{x} = .78$ | $\bar{x} = .78$ | $\bar{x} = .74$ | $\bar{x} = .76$ | $\bar{x} = .90$ |

**TABLE 7-3  Ratings of attachment behaviors in normal (control) and prepsychotic (index) infants and their mothers**

| Group | Feeding | | | | Holding | | | | Touching | | | |
|---|---|---|---|---|---|---|---|---|---|---|---|---|
| | N | Mean | sd | t | N | Mean | sd | t | N | Mean | sd | t |
| Infant | 19 | | | | 28 | | | | 28 | | | |
| Control | 11 | 3.50 | .531 | .450 | 14 | 3.10 | .415 | 1.46 | 14 | 3.25 | .476 | 1.11 |
| Index | 8 | 3.35 | .826 | | 14 | 2.75 | .792 | | 14 | 2.90 | .588 | |
| Mother | 19 | | | | 28 | | | | 28 | | | |
| Control | 11 | 4.00 | .512 | .656 | 14 | 3.45 | .652 | 3.23** | 14 | 3.50 | .451 | 3.54*** |
| Index | 8 | 3.75 | .985 | | 14 | 2.75 | .487 | | 14 | 2.75 | .662 | |

| Group | Eye-gazing | | | | Affect | | | |
|---|---|---|---|---|---|---|---|---|
| | N | Mean | sd | t | N | Mean | sd | t |
| Infant | 28 | | | | 28 | | | |
| Control | 14 | 3.25 | .851 | .434 | 14 | 3.75 | .853 | 3.92*** |
| Index | 14 | 2.70 | .993 | | 14 | 2.50 | .821 | |
| Mother | 28 | | | | 28 | | | |
| Control | 14 | 3.75 | .416 | 2.53* | 14 | 4.20 | .628 | 3.52*** |
| Index | 14 | 3.25 | .615 | | 14 | 3.25 | .795 | |

*p .01
**p .005
***p .001

mothers and infants. For this global assessment, the three judges looked at the film footage for each index and control case in random order, and then responded to a series of questions (e.g., "Does this mother/infant seem healthy . . . strongly attached . . . avoiding . . . content . . . distressed?"). Without knowing the identity of the cases, one of the investigators sorted the responses into three categories that were given a numerical value on an ordinal scale:

1 = negative responses (e.g., avoiding, not healthy)
2 = neutral responses (e.g., healthy, content)
3 = strongly positive responses (e.g., strongly attached)

## Results

Mean ratings were determined by taking the average of the three raters for each of four film segments for the variables of holding, touching, eye gaze, and affect, and for each of the three segments for the variable of feeding in cases where sufficient feeding scenes were available. T-tests determined whether the observed differences between means were significant. One-tailed tests of significance were used, with t values significant at less than .01.

The findings are summarized in Table 7-3. The trends of overall ratings in each of the categories—feeding, holding, touching, eye gaze, and affect—went to the predicted direction. The means of both infant and maternal behaviors in all variables in the control group are consistently higher than those of the index group.

*Infant Findings* When t-tests were used to compare normal infants with prepsychotic infants, no significant difference between groups was observed in feeding behavior, touching, holding, eye gaze. For affect, however, infants in the control group showed significantly higher levels (p < .001) of pleasurable emotional expressiveness and responsiveness than infants in the prepsychotic group.

It was then post hoc hypothesized that the lumping of all of the index infants into one diagnostic grouping—early childhood psychosis—might have obscured some significant differences in the categories of touching, holding, and eye gaze, which initially appeared to have no significant differences between index and control families. Thus the index group was divided into those subsequently diagnosed as autistic (N = 9) and those suffering other forms of early childhood psychosis (Symbiotic Psychosis of Childhood, and Mixed Form of

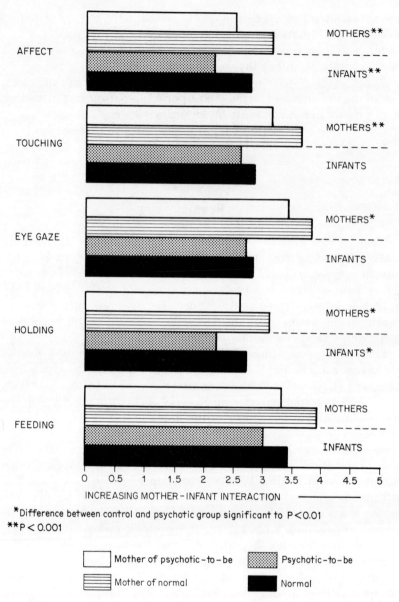

*Difference between control and psychotic group significant to P<0.01
**P < 0.001

Figure 7.1   Mean ratings of strength of responsiveness in first six months of life of control (normal) group of infants and mothers, and group of infants-to-become psychotic and their mothers.

Early Childhood Psychosis) (N = 5). T-tests were calculated between these two groupings of the index cases. For touching and holding, there was no significant difference among groups, indicating a homogeneity of those behaviors in the total index sample. However, for eye gaze there was a significant difference between the subsequently autistic children and those suffering other forms of childhood psychosis (p < .01). The autistic children avoided more and initiated less eye contact with their mothers than did other ill children. It followed that this significant difference in eye gaze also distinguished the subsequently autistic children and control children (p > .01). For the infants subsequently diagnosed as having other forms of childhood psychosis, there was no significant difference in eye gaze in the first six months of life when compared to normal group infants.

*Mother Findings*  For the two groups of mothers, there was no significant difference in feeding. However, mothers of control infants achieved significantly higher ratings for holding (p < .005), touching (p < .001), eye gaze (p < .01), and affect (p < .001). Thus, in the two categories of holding and touching, the two groups of infants were not distinguished, even controlling for subsequent diagnosis, whereas there were significant differences between mothers of prepsychotic and normal infants indicative of greater reciprocity, responsiveness, initiative, and less avoidance and withdrawal in these bonding/attachment parameters.

*General Impressions of Attachment*  After the investigator sorted the raters' "general impressions of attachment" into three categories, the values for each case were averaged. A mean of 2 to 3 was considered indicative of normal attachment, a mean of 1 to 1.667 was considered poor attachment. Each mother and child in the normal and prepsychotic groups was assigned to a cell, representing either normal or poor attachment. Of the control group, three infants appeared to be poorly attached and eleven appeared to be normally attached. Of the index group, eight infants appeared to be poorly attached and six appeared to be normally attached. A Chi-square test with Yates correction for small sample size was computed. There were no significant differences between the general impressions of attachment of the two groups. On the other hand, with regard to the mothers, eleven index mothers appeared poorly attached and three normally attached; in the control group, twelve mothers appeared normally attached and two mothers appeared poorly attached. This distribution was significantly different from chance (p < .01).

## Discussion

This study was illuminating in several important ways. The difference in affect between control and index mothers and between control and index infants was striking. This confirmed our earlier clinical impressions of subdued but nonetheless genuine emotional avoidance or dampening in the first six months of life for both mothers and babies in the prepsychotic group. From this we can speculate on different levels.

For the infant there may be a tendency toward dampened or unresponsive affect that may be the result of an innate predisposition which may, in turn, influence maternal affect. Thus a fretful, fearful, or unresponsive infant might greatly influence the reciprocity of the mother-child interaction.

Where the mother is depressed, her internal preoccupation may lead to unresponsiveness to the infant who may then cease attempting to communicate with the mother. Further, overstimulating, frustrating, or confusingly inconsistent or paradoxical parental actions may lead the infant to attempt to ward off the parent through avoiding contact. Each of these pathways appeared in one or more of the case studies in Chapter 6. Although the research data illustrates these complex pathways through which infant and maternal moods influence each other, it does not confirm causal connections with the subsequent appearance of childhood illness. Nonetheless, the importance of reciprocal responsiveness and mutual entrainment into social behavior by both mother and infant in the earliest months of a baby's life should not be underestimated.

It is interesting to note that feeding differences do not emerge for the two groups, since psychoanalytic theory has traditionally focused on the oral phase of libidinal development. However, as the review in Chapter 3 of the findings of contemporary infancy research shows, additional modalities of physical contact and eye gaze may be as important to the vicissitudes of early development as the actual feeding. Thus, aversion and unresponsiveness in touching, holding, or looking may occur more frequently and be more crucially traumatic than maternal feeding interferences. This, of course, does not vitiate the developmental principle that underlies the oral libidinal phase (Freud, 1905, 1926): that the infant's heightened state of organismic tension, which is initially experienced as a primitive life-and-death anxiety, must be soothed so that the infant can gradually incorporate, internalize, and ultimately identify with a mother who is experienced as primarily gratifying. However, in the more modern concept, the infant experiences organismic tension more broadly through his body. Contemporary infancy research, which emphasizes other modalities of communication in addition to feeding, shifts, as Bowlby (1969) has done, away from a unitary concept of orality. He posits, in his studies of attachment, a group of behaviors—babbling, holding, touching, eye gaze, and eating. Reciprocally, the mother can frustrate or consummate the infant's attempts for gratification in any of these attachment modalities that are instinctually determined for both mother and baby. Furthermore, feeding may sometimes bring out the best in a mother since it is a more clearly structured situation than other social interactions that highlight other aspects of the attachment.

Another important finding of this study is in the modalities of holding and touching (proximal forms of interaction) and in the modality of eye gaze (a distal form of interaction). For touching and holding, we see significant differences between control and index mothers, but not between the infants. This suggests that maternal aversion or unresponsiveness in these modalities can be pathogenic to the child. For the prepsychotic and normal infants in this study, the lack of significant differences in touching and holding indicates the readiness of both groups of babies to engage in proximal (close bodily) communication with their mothers in early life, a capacity that can be thwarted or facilitated by the parent.

With regard to eye gaze, it is interesting that while there is not an overall significant difference between children of the index and control groups, pre-autistic babies initiate less gazing and avoid more eye contact with their mothers than either prepsychotic infants of other classifications or normal controls. We know from studies reviewed in Chapter 3 that early reciprocal eye gaze is important in facilitating normal development. But in the autistic infants this is impaired—whether because of an inborn disturbance or secondary to an interactional failure with the caretaker. As a consequence, it is possible that very rapidly pre-autistic children are handicapped by the development of a lower perceptual capacity for distal interaction with inanimate and animate objects in their environment.

Perception, especially as mediated by vision, has a key function normally as growth ensues in the development of higher levels of communication and in the psychologic process of internalization of parental images. But once ill, autistic children are stunted in communication and interaction in a way that supports the idea of distal perceptual interferences. They relate to objects often by holding them close to their faces and manipulating them in stereotypic, often nonfunctional repetitive ways. Likewise, autistic children do not for the most part communicate adequately with other people. The other prepsychotic children who were not autistic were closer to the control group means in their social use of vision. Consistent with this, they generally achieved as time passed more normal distal capacities for relating (speaking, playing with objects, facial expression) than autistic children. However, like autistic children they remained deficient in areas of psychologic develoment that are grounded in early proximal reciprocal mother-infant interactions—the capacity to modulate emotional closeness and separateness.

## Conclusion

Although the data base has been small, the results from the controlled and blind study of the infancy home movies supported the earlier clinical descriptions of family interaction. It was gratifying that earlier investigators of the films had not been led astray by their knowledge of the subsequent diagnoses of the children. In terms of the overall development of The Early Natural History of Childhood Psychosis Project, there has been progress toward generating an etiological theory of psychotic disturbances in early childhood. The initial case studies led to hypotheses of specific kinds of failures in mother-infant bonding which were systematically tested with the methodology reported in this chapter. Likewise, the case studies also led to the empirical study of cognitive development in infancy in index and control groups that is reported in the next chapter.

Both the clinical studies as well as the empirical efforts lead to more refined hypotheses concerning aberrant and normal intrapsychic growth which go beyond the basic understanding of bonding parameters and the reciprocal nature of their influence on emotional attachment. Bringing all of this information together—in the light of contemporary research on infancy and childhood psychosis—is the work of Chapters 9 and 10.

# Chapter 8

# A Piagetian-Based Analysis of Intellectual Development from Birth to Two Years in Subsequently Psychotic Children

Another productive avenue of exploration has been the study of the early cognitive development, as categorized by Piaget's stages of sensorimotor development, of the group of children premorbid for childhood psychosis and an equal number of control cases. This had appeared to be a valuable avenue of research since, from the time of Bleuler's work (1911), psychosis and cognition have been inextricably linked in descriptive and explanatory models. As we saw earlier, in the field of childhood psychosis beginning with the work of Despert (1941), Kanner (1946), and Bender (1947), researchers have universally considered the profound disorders of speech and thinking to be critical diagnostic functions of childhood psychosis. Bender and Freedman (1952) have shown that unevenness seen in the different spheres of ego functioning in psychotic children frequently began in infancy. In addition, Anthony (1956, 1958) has shown with empirical observations and tests of psychotic children beyond the toddler stage that an absence of object permanence and the presence of infantile sensorimotor cognitive behavior patterns was found in these children. However, because Anthony was studying older children, he was not able to determine whether these problems represented developmental failures in the first two years of life or regressions from more advanced intellectual attainments.

Our film data of the infancies of the subsequently psychotic children provided the opportunity to view the course of early intellectual development to see when the index cases deviated from normal—if at all. Further, it gives the investigators the vantage point of viewing cognition in its earliest stages, before the libidinal, object relational, and intellectual lines of development become so intertwined as to make it impossible to tease apart the hypothesized etiological factors of psychosis. Since this phase of our study is descriptive clinical analysis, we did not have well-defined hypotheses regarding the cognitive functioning in childhood psychosis. It was possible that primitive cognitive deficits were primary etiological factors of childhood psychosis. Alternatively, other aspects of the psychosis may lead to failures in intellectual growth. From the clinical vantage point, description of the cognitive capabilities of children who later became psychotic could be correlated with the Childhood Psychosis Project's findings of the initial signs and symptoms of the illness and the patterns of the mother-infant interaction. Our work was guided by two questions. First, how do intellectual capacities develop in children with childhood psychosis as compared with normal children? Secondly, how do cognitive capacities differ, if at all, in children with different kinds of childhood psychosis?

The choice of a Piagetian-based approach for this study grew out of two considerations—one empirical, and one theoretical. The empirical consideration related to the nature of our data base. While the home movies of the index cases provided prospective data before the signs and symptoms of the illness appeared, data which was generated in a naturalistic setting without the artifacts of the experimental situation, the movies lacked any kind of standardization. We have varying amounts of film from different time periods in the early lives of the children. However, these empirical limitations can be seen as parallel to Piaget's own naturalistic approach in studying cognitive development in early infancy through observing his own children (1936). Additionally, Piagetian categories have been adapted for studies employing naturalistic observation, such as Chevalier-Skolnikoff's application to primatology research (1977). Second, Piagetian theory is congruent with contemporary research findings concerning the mental capacities of the infant. Such research focuses on the capabilities of the neonate in areas of perception, cognition, the establishment of a sense of self, and the beginnings of social contacts between self and others, and it often shows infants to be more sophisticated in these areas than previously believed.

We chose to focus on the sensorimotor period for several reasons. It is completed by twenty-four months of age in the normal course of development. Its completion is marked by the toddler's new capacity for symbolic representations of objects and events. Its end also marks an important convergence of the developmental lines of the cognitive capacity for symbolic representation and the affective capacity for libidinal object constancy. Clinically, by twenty-four months of age the majority of index cases had developed clear signs and symptoms of psychopathology, so that etiological clues could be most productively sought prior to the first two years of life. Sensorimotor behaviors categorize those aspects of intelligence which are expressed through the child's actions on himself and objects in the world—they are the primitive anlage of "intelligence,"expressed through motoric actions. Such behaviors could be clearly observed in soundless home movies.

According to Piaget, sensorimotor intelligence is "that aspect of intelligence which is a preparation in the field of elementary activity for what will much later become the operations of reflective thought" (1945). In the beginning of the sensorimotor period, from approximately birth to four weeks, the infant does not involve itself in the world of objects. However, as soon as the habits of grasping are acquired, the formation of the object concept is put into motion. Objects become, over the course of the first two years of life, things which are "conceived as permanent, substantial, external to the self, and firm in existence even though they do not directly affect perception" (Piaget, 1937). Even with changes in position, objects maintain their identity. In the stages of the sensorimotor period, the infant moves from an objectless state to an egocentric mode of relating to objects, to a highly elaborated development of the object concept. In this final stage, the child is able to recognize the existence of objects apart from his own actions on them, as well as to be able mentally to represent external objects and patterns of his own actions upon these objects. Table 8-1 provides, in summary form, descriptions and examples of the six stages of sensorimotor development.

## Methodology

The three investigators viewed all of the movies of the fourteen index cases and the fourteen control cases (see Table 7-1 for a demographic summary of the families). The procedure for assigning

**TABLE 8-1    Characteristics of the sensorimotor intelligence series as manifested by human infants***

| Stage | Description | Major distinguishing behavioral parameters | Example |
|---|---|---|---|
| 1<br>Reflex<br>0–1 months | Involuntary responses occurring without cerebral cortex participation. | Involuntary. | Rooting and sucking. |
| 2<br>Primary circular reaction<br>1–4 months | An infant's action that is centered on his own body, and which he learns to repeat in order to reinstate the event. | Repetitive coordinations of own body. Acquired adaptations. Recognizes various objects and contexts. | Repeated hand-hand clasping. Conditioned reflexes. |
| 3<br>Secondary circular reaction<br>4–10 months | Repeated ("circular") attempts to re-produce environmental ("secondary") events initially discovered by chance. | Environment oriented behaviors. Establishment of relationships between objects and actions. Semi-intentional (an initial act is not intentional but subsequent one is). | Swings object and attends to the swinging spectacle or to the resultant sound. Repeats. Smiles and brightens at mother's face or voice. |

168

| | | |
|---|---|---|
| 4<br>Coordination of secondary behaviors<br>10–12 months | Two or more independent behavioral acts become intercoordinated, one serving as instrument to another. | Intentional; goal established from outset; establishment of relationship between two objects which are explored as well as acted upon; familiar behaviors applied to new situations. | Setting aside an obstacle in order to obtain an object behind it; can pull a cord to get a bell to ring ("gets the connection"). |
| 5<br>Tertiary circular reaction<br>12–18 months | The child becomes curious about an object or person's functions and actions, and object-object and object-force relationships. Trial-and-error experimentation. | Behavior becomes variable and not stereotyped. Interest in novelty for its own sake. Coordination of object-space relationships. Begins to see others as autonomous. | Experimentally discovering that one object, such as a stick, can be used to obtain another object. |
| 6<br>Invention of new means<br>18–24 months | The solution is arrived at mentally, and not through trial-and error experimentation. | The child can represent objects and events not present symbolically. | Mentally figuring out how one object can be used to obtain another object. |

*From Chevalier-Skolnikoff (1976).

sensorimotor ratings follows. It is important to note that the methodology is of a clinical nature, utilizing agreements reached through conference.

*1. Identification of Behavior* Whenever a child was observed performing an action upon the environment, or engaged in self-manipulation, the film was stopped. If the three raters agreed by conference that this was an activity that was captured on the film with sufficient clarity to rate, they proceeded to step 2 below. Otherwise the film was continued.

*2. Determination of the Child's Age* The age of the child in the segment to be rated was ascertained from film markings, anniversaries such as holidays and birthdays, parents' recall, and visualization of gross motor-development milestones, with the availability of the child's pediatric records to aid in verifying such milestones. These aids, in addition to the researchers' backgrounds in clinical and developmental research, led to a high degree of agreement as to the age of the child in the segments that were studied.

*3. Rating of Sensorimotor Stage* The identified segment was viewed several times, often using slow-motion and single-frame projection. A conference rating of the specific sensorimotor stage indexing the behavior being enacted by the child was then determined. Table 8-2 provides an example of the kinds of behaviors which appeared in the home movies of one of the index cases.

## Findings

The data is summarized in Table 8-3 for the index group and Table 8-4 for the control group. For both groups, the following information is provided for each subject: a subject identification which is congruent with reports of other phases of the Project in other chapters to assist the reader in cross-referencing data;[1] the age range of the subject appearing in the film; the total number of behaviors assigned sensorimotor ratings; the number of age-appropriate behaviors—

---

[1] Cases 2 and 7 in Chapter 6 could not be included in this study because their films were no longer available. Thirteen cases listed in Table 8-3 received blind ratings of mother-infant interactions (Chapter 7). One case was a new addition to this phase of the Project.

**TABLE 8-2** *Example of behaviors and sensorimotor ratings of an index case*
Case: S.I.
Diagnosis: Autism

| Observed behavior | Age of child | Sensorimotor stage |
|---|---|---|
| Smiles and brightens at mother's face and voice. | 5 months | Stage 3 |
| Fingers, looks at, and puts shoe in mouth. | 12 months | Stage 2 |
| Holds jar and touches it without visual accompaniment. | 24 months | Stage 2 |
| Watches an adult push plunger on toy top, and then repeatedly does so himself. | 28 months | Stage 4 |

those behaviors which appeared at the chronologically normative time; and the percentage of age-appropriate behaviors, which was determined by dividing column 4 by column 3, thereby making the data among subjects comparable. It is important to note that lower stages exist contemporaneously with the age-appropriate stages without being indicative of pathology. For example, a stage-4 behavior at eleven months is age appropriate, although stage-3 behaviors may also be present. The next column shows the highest sensorimotor stage reached during the filmed period up to the subject's second year of life. For the index group, the next column provides the diagnosis. We divide the index-group children into two diagnostic categories—autism and early childhood psychosis. Early childhood psychosis subsumes those children suffering from symbiotic psychosis of childhood and the mixed form of early childhood psychosis, as outlined in Chapter 2.

The final column of Table 8-3 provides the highest sensorimotor stage reached for the index cases in the first forty-one months of life. The extended period of observation for the index cases maximized the number of observations for each child and also provided a window into the cognitive development after the sensorimotor stages would have been completed. The findings indicate that some of the subsequently psychotic children did not complete progression through the sensorimotor stages by twenty-four months, but later showed evidence of higher stages of behavior. Others remained fixated at the level of functioning achieved in the first two years, and there is the suggestion that regressions in intellectual functioning may occur after the second year of life. The observations of the control group were not extended beyond the second year of life, since each subject for whom there was data available up to twenty-four months displayed stage-6 behavior.

*Differences Between Index and Control Groups*    Comparing the data in Tables 8-3 and 8-4, the following findings emerge:

1. All of the control cases evidenced behaviors of the normatively appropriate sensorimotor stage in the movie footage provided. Further, the five control cases for whom there is footage up to twenty-four months of age show at least one behavior at sensorimotor stage 6. This compares with the index group, where only one case demonstrated stage-6 sensorimotor behavior by twenty-four months.

2. A striking finding is the difference in total number of sensorimotor behaviors observed in the control and index groups, especially if it is examined in relation to the differing age range of observations available for each group. For the control group there was a total of 138 behaviors observed in a period spanning 167 months. This is compared to the 73 behaviors of the index group, spanning an observational period of 267 months.[2] Thus although the data base is unstandardized, it is apparent that there are more behaviors observed in the control group. It appears, therefore, that the normal children are more active with objects in their environment.

3. In comparing the percentage of age-appropriate behaviors between control and index groups, a Z Test for Differences in Percentages was used. The null hypothesis of no difference was rejected (Z = 3.82, p < .001). This indicated a significant difference between age-appropriate behaviors in the index and control groups. Thus we find that there are also more *age-appropriate* behaviors in the control children than in the index group.

*Clinical Findings.*    The second question which guided this study was how cognitive capacities differ, if at all, in children with different

---

[2]This information is included for descriptive purposes only. Tests of difference were not computed because the data does not lend itself to these calculations.

types of childhood psychosis. Close examination of the data in Table 8-3 reveals some interesting trends which provide a background against which this question can be productively considered. Three patterns emerge in the cognitive development of the subsequently psychotic children. First, there are those subjects who progress through the usual course of sensorimotor stages, but at a slower rate than normal children, which we shall call *"cognitive slowing."* The second group includes those who progress through the first three stages and show at least one behavior at sensorimotor stage 4, but whose overall functioning appears limited to stages 2 and 3. This particular group appears to demonstrate what will be termed a *"cognitive arrest"*—the first stages of sensorimotor intelligence appear, but no further development ensues. The third group is composed of those subjects whose capacities are *"cognitively fixated"* at the most primitive levels, showing a preponderance of stage-2 behaviors.

The subjects in the first or slowed group—F.D., C.H., and Amy—evidence progression through the stages of sensorimotor development at a slower rate than what is normative. Subject C.H. showed stage-6 behavior at eighteen months of age; F.D. showed stage-6 behavior at twenty-nine months; and Amy was at stage 5 at twenty-four months. Of these children, C.H. and Amy had the highest percentage of age-appropriate behaviors (.75 and .57 respectively) of the index group. Diagnostically, F.D. is autistic but with moderate relatedness, and C.H. and Amy suffer one of the other psychoses of early childhood.

The subjects in the cognitive arrest group—Joan, Edward, S.I., S.H., S.Q., and Q.E.—all show some, albeit limited, capacity for stage-4 behavior, with the majority of the behaviors being at stages 2 and 3. This indicates attainment of the beginning of object permanence and the ability to act with intentionality; however, the majority of their behaviors are still body-centered and involve trial-and-error manipulations of the world of objects. They do not show an ability by the age of twenty-four months to endow objects with a reality of their own, which is a hallmark of stage 5. Only one subject, S.H., showed one instance of stage-5 behavior at thirty-six months. Diagnostically, this group is mixed: Joan, S.I., S.Q. and Q.E. are autistic, while Edward and S.H. are diagnosed as suffering another form of early childhood psychosis.

The third, or primitive fixation group consists of subjects demonstrating the lowest level of cognitive development. Two distinct

**TABLE 8-3** *Summary of findings for index group*

| Case | Observations | Total no. observations | No. age-appropriate | Percentage observations age-appropriate | Highest stage reached during sensorimotor period (0–24 months) | Diagnosis | Further stage reached in first 3½ years |
|---|---|---|---|---|---|---|---|
| C.H. | 5–18 months | 4 | 3 | .75 | 6 | Early Child-hood Psychosis | — |
| Amy S. | 4–24 months | 7 | 4 | .57 | 5 | Early Child-hood Psychosis | — |
| S.H. | 4–36 months | 6 | 2 | .33 | 3 | Early Child-hood Psychosis | 5 (at 36 months) |
| Edward P. | 4–24 months | 3 | 1 | .33 | 4 | Early Child-hood Psychosis | — |
| F.D. | 6–36 months | 6 | 2 | .33 | 4 | Autism | 6 (at 29 months) |

| | | | | | | | |
|---|---|---|---|---|---|---|---|
| Jean | 2–18 months | 6 | 2 | .33 | 3 | Autism | — |
| Joan L. | 4–24 months | 7 | 2 | .29 | 4 | Autism | — |
| S.I. | 5–28 months | 4 | 1 | .25 | 3 | Autism | 4 (at 28 months) |
| Ethan C. | 5–41 months | 6 | 1 | .17 | 3 | Early Child- hood Psychosis | 3 (at 41 months) |
| Q.E. | 12–36 months | 6 | 0 | .00 | 4 | Autism | 4 (at 36 months) |
| Robert N. | 33–36 months | 2 | 0 | .00 | — | Autism | 4 (at 36 months) |
| S.Q. | 7–36 months | 6 | 0 | .00 | 3 | Autism | 4 (at 36 months) |
| Steven O. | 5–12 months | 3 | 0 | .00 | 2 | Autism | — |
| Ken Y. | 6–12 months | 3 | 0 | .00 | 2 | Autism | — |

**TABLE 8-4  Summary of findings for control group**

| Case | Age range of observations | Total no. observations | No. age appropriate | Percentage of observations age-appropriate | Highest sensorimotor stage reached during filmed periods in the first 24 months |
|------|---------------------------|------------------------|---------------------|--------------------------------------------|----------------------------------------------------------------------------------|
| A | 4 months–2years | 12 | 9 | .75 | 6 |
| S | 4 months–10 months | 8 | 4 | .50 | 4 |
| F | 8 months–2½ years | 10 | 4 | .40 | 6 |
| BB | 6 weeks–2 years | 15 | 9 | .60 | 6 |
| J | 1 month–6 months | 5 | 2 | .40 | 2 |
| CC | 2 months–6 months | 4 | 1 | .25 | 2 |
| L | 4 months–1 year | 10 | 7 | .70 | 5 |
| KK | 4 months–2 years | 15 | 8 | .53 | 6 |
| N | 2 weeks–6 months | 9 | 6 | .67 | 3 |
| LL | 4 months–1 year | 8 | 4 | .50 | 4 |
| $P_1$ | 2 months–6 months | 10 | 2 | .25 | 3 |
| TT | 0– 2 years | 15 | 10 | .67 | 6 |
| $P_2$ | 3 months–6 months | 7 | 3 | .43 | 3 |
| XX | 2 months–10 months | 10 | 7 | .70 | 4 |

clinical configurations comprise this group. The first consists of Ken and Steven, both of whom show no behaviors above stage 2 by the age of twelve months. The second group consists of Jean and Ethan who show very early age-appropriate actions (at two and three months for Jean, and at eight months for Ethan); however, there appears to be a fixation at stages 2 and 3 for both subjects. Diagnostically, Ken, Steven, and Jean were classified as autistic and Ethan was in the early childhood psychosis group with the psychiatric records noting some autistic features as well. The probable fixation of these four cases at sensorimotor stages 2 and 3 suggests that these children remained through the first three years of life in a cognitive state in which body-centered actions predominate, with little sense of distinction between the self and objects in the outside world.

Descriptively, it appeared that the prepsychotic children who achieve the highest level of intellectual functioning in the first two years of life generally are in the category of early childhood psychosis (which subsumes symbiotic psychosis of childhood and mixed form of early childhood psychosis) while the majority of those who are primitively fixated are autistic. To test this hypothesis of the relationship between diagnostic classification and the three postulated patterns of early cognitive development in the index cases, a 2-by-3 contingency table was constructed and the Chi-square statistic calculated. This classification of diagnostic category by cognitive group yielded a Chi-square of .932 (df = 3) which was not statistically significant.

Another clinical question which would be interesting to investigate is that of cognitive regression. Unfortunately, the home movie data does not provide an appropriate empirical base from which to attempt to answer such a question. There is not enough film footage beyond the first two years of life to see whether regressions in cognitive functioning occur with any regularity in the index cases. If it were available, this data could be used to add validity to Anthony's postulation of "the regression of the object concept" which he derived from the experimental study of older psychotic children (1958). There is one case in the index group which seems to show a regression in cognitive function. This is S.I., an autistic boy who achieved stage 3 appropriately at age five months, as evidenced by brightening at his mother's face and voice. He then appeared to fall back to stage-2 behaviors, and progress only reappeared in the third year when he showed a stage-4 sensorimotor behavior.

## Discussion

In this substudy of the Childhood Psychosis Project, it is important to emphasize the limitations of our data base which affect the kinds of inferences that can be made from this study. There were a different number of ratable segments for each child, and unlike the experimental situation where the subjects are present to elicit optimal responses, we could not be certain if what was observed was truly the child's optimal cognitive capacity. The absence of a higher-stage behavior cannot be taken as firm evidence of the child's incapacity to attain it under other circumstances. Nonetheless, some important conclusions can be drawn from the investigation. On a descriptive level, there emerged three patterns of intellectual development in the prepsychotic children—primitive fixation, arrest, and slowed development. Although with the limited number of cases these patterns were not statistically correlated with particular pathologic diagnoses, discussed in relation to specific case material they were of heuristic value in generating hypotheses for future testing.

The most striking finding from the analysis was the statistically significant higher percentage of age-appropriate sensorimotor behaviors in the control as compared to the index group. In this regard other writers (Despert, 1941; Bender, 1947, 1952) have pointed toward a poorly integrated development of locomotor, fine motor, and visual motor skills, resulting in erratic patterns of functioning. The unevenness in motor development and the many lines of developmental delay of ego functions could partially account for the significantly fewer number of acitivities observed in the prepsychotic group of children. The paucity of behaviors may also derive to some extent from the kinds of parental withdrawal and disruption of infant response that have been described in Chapters 6 and 7. Thus Greenspan (1979) suggests that when parents are absent, depressed, or fail to provide an ambience that is active, stimulating, and consistent from the point of view of interpersonal animate and inanimate object interaction, a child may have traumatic or insufficient sensory stimulation to develop an optimum or developmentally progressive and multiplying number of action schema. Such a hypothesis leads to the additional and interconnected speculation that the inactivity of prepsychotic infants may also be partially caused by failures of the children to emotionally cathect the animate and inanimate object worlds. This would occur in the babies secondary to their being inadequately entrained into the world, or to defensive withdrawal from inchoate and traumatic parenting, or to organic disabilities that lead to avoidance or incapacity to interact with environmental stimulation.

Further, it is useful to make some inferential generalizations as to how these prepsychotic children may cognitively and affectively experience their own bodies and their worlds. Thus the primitively fixated children—who were mostly autistic—gave the qualitative impression that they were in a vacuum, as it were, with inutile hands, failed language, and fragmented, undeveloped affects. They appeared to be no more able to interact on inanimate objects in their environment than with people. The profound and global nature of their syndrome distinguished it from the other pictures of childhood psychosis. A further note on this group is that the autoeroticisms and stereotypies such as the rocking and hand flapping of the autistic children are also categorizable as stage-2 behaviors since they are purely body-centered. In connection with this, these fixated children continued to show a large percentage of primary circular reactions, such as bringing objects to their mouths, well into the third year of life. Normal children on occasion show behaviors characteristic of an intellectual stage that they have long surpassed, but these behaviors are the exceptions in contrast to the ubiquitousness of primitive activities in the first group of children. In addition, both the primitively fixated infants and the children who were somewhat later arrested in sensorimotor cognitive development may be understood to not gain the normal sense in their second year of life that they can act with intentionality in the world and have a foreseen effect on people and things.

In conclusion, it appears that primitive mental stage fixations and developmental lags occur in the first two years of life of children who will later be diagnosed as suffering a psychosis of early childhood. One has the impression that such a child may remain in a world without objects where images appear and vanish seemingly, to the infant, as a result of his own activities. The concept of an object as having a reality separate from himself does not exist. For some of the subsequently ill babies, more slowly than normal, objects may ultimately gain permanence, substantiality, and an identity that is not a function of the baby himself; the child's body may, if progress occurs, become an object in itself among the world of other objects that will have an existence apart from the child's immediate perception of them.

When fixation and retardation occur, it is generally contemporaneous with the appearance of the other affective, interpersonal behavioral, and motoric signs and symptoms of childhood psychosis described in detail in Chapter 6. We cannot determine, however, to what extent cognitive deficits are a contributing factor to, a consequence of, or a codetermining factor in the illness. Likewise, it is not possible to pinpoint how much and in what instances neurologic dysfunction may contribute to the overall picture of impaired intellectual and emotional growth.

With more refined methodologies for assessing infants at risk for childhood psychosis, longitudinal studies can be carried out in which there will be more formal testing of the cognitive capacities in conjunction with assessment of psychological structuralization of children as they develop. Such studies hold the possibility of testing the hypotheses and inferences which this section of the Childhood Psychosis Project has generated.

*Chapter 9*

# A Summary of the Findings of the Early Natural History of Childhood Psychosis Study: Toward an Etiological Theory

The investigation of the early natural history of childhood psychosis resembles in a way trying to paddle a canoe out of a swamp. Many promising currents and flows of water run through the pockets of grass and islands, but some dry up, and others seem to go in circles. Only a few converge at the far side of the swamp to form a river that moves on its way. So too with research: some promising ideas dry up, and some leads seem to grow stronger and reinforce each other, advancing our understanding of the phenomenon being explored. Our investigation has paralleled this course; and in this chapter we first review the paths the Childhood Psychosis Project has traversed and the concrete findings that have emerged, then we begin to examine these findings in search of meaningful correlations. These are the converging currents that lead one downstream and point the way to advancing our conceptualization of both aberrant infancy phenomena in childhood psychosis and normal infancy development.

Findings in the Project fall into three categories—observations of behavior, psychological formulations, and historical information. The *observations of behavior* comprise the documentation of the social interactions in which parents and infants engage, the recording of the earliest symptoms of childhood psychosis, and the unfolding of the behaviors that indicated cognitive capacity in the first two years of life in the prepsychotic and normal children. *Psychological formulations* include our understanding of intrapsychic conflicts and impulses that led parents to their behaviors, as gleaned from the psychotherapies of the parents. It also includes our attempts to construct the intrapsychic experience of the children. The category of *historical information* pulls together medical information pertinent to potential organic disturbances, and discusses the initial history and later course of illness in the children.

## Observations of Behavior

### Social Interactions

Our study of the behavior of parents and children provided both descriptive and statistical data which were consistent with each other and mutually reinforcing. Close analysis of the process of mother-infant behavior led to the following generalizations. There were disturbances in the pattern of mother-infant behavior, often in the first six months of life, in families where a child subsequently developed one of the syndromes of childhood psychosis. One could say that there was often a "dampened" responsiveness between mother and infant in which sometimes the parent seemed to be the primary contributor and at other times the infant. But far more than this, it is possible to specify how dampened response is in effect an omission, muting, or thwarting of one or more of the interactive behaviors that occur between a mother and baby, again with parent, child, or sometimes even both being the important contributors to the problem. So we see families in which there was a disturbance in one or several of the bonding modalities of maternal holding, infant clinging, touching, gazing, vocalizing, affective interchange, and feeding.

It is possible to go beyond this descriptive level with the recognition that the bonding problems are characterized by a range of patterns for which the adjectives "thwarting," "dampening." and "omission" are not adequate. The study showed that there are often qualitative and quantitative as well as multidimensional problems. Thus the *rhythm* of the interactions between parent and child were frequently out of synchrony with each other so that at times a child required a more rapid or slower tempo of response from a parent to allow contact to take place. Additionally, the *physical force* of a parental action was seen in some cases to be too powerful to allow (or encourage) the infant to make an organized response. At other times when a child's response was slow and weak, mothers in our series were similarly slow, physically timid, and affectively lifeless, so that little occurred in the dyad. A more animated parent might have been able to draw these infants into an interpersonal engagement. In the series of cases, the parents and infants seemed most often to be engaged in a timid or awkwardly choreographed dance.

Generically, across the series of index cases there was a failure for attachment to be consummated in one or more of its modalities. Consummation is an important concept which is likely to have significant developmental implications. It may be defined as the series of actions and psychological states that occur when the mother or the baby has an impulse toward or seeks contact with the other person. The impulse may unfold, for example, through touching, holding or being held, and/or through smiling and the smile being returned. When the impulse is not met or reciprocated, it cannot be consummated, so that organismically tension is heightened and a psychological attachment does not ensue, leaving in its wake various states of dysphoria. Dysphoria could sometimes be observed on the faces of the parents or infants when their impulses were thwarted as discrete affects of confusion, dejection, apathy, depression, and anger.

From the series of index and control cases in the project there emerge five general categories and nine specific patterns of parent-infant behavior that impede interactive consummations of affective states, reciprocity, and bonding.

**TABLE 9-1**   *General categories of disburbed parent-infant behavior*

*1. Adequate parenting and an unresponsive child*

In this configuration, parents may be adequately responsive and even as nurturing as the most responsive of control-group mothers. However, their infants are subdued, if not at times lifeless. As time passes, unrewarded by their baby, the parents become increasingly anxious, inconsistent, contradictory, and sometimes angry in their behavior.

*2. Parenting characterized by stiffness, slow, and partial response, and lack of maternal animation and molding across the bonding modalities, coupled with a similarly lifeless and unresponsive child*

However, there are no specific distortions or omissions of response on the part of either mother or baby.

*3. Maternal care which establishes a particular pattern of dismutual reponse with*

**TABLE 9-1** *General category of disturbed parent-infant behavior* (continued)
*the infant through paradoxical stimulation and avoidance of the baby, and an initially responsive baby*

The mother of Joan (Case 1) gave the clearest example of this in nuzzling the child's cheek so that the baby smiled and turned to look at her, but then avoiding the infant's gaze. Thus the mother gave the child contradictory messages to look at her and not to look at her. This was a form of kinesically rather than verbally delivered double bind. Consummation of the pleasurable affect that the mother aroused in the child through nuzzling did not occur since shared gazing and smiling were thwarted. This particular configuration involved eye-gaze; however, a similar pattern may occur in other bonding modalities.

*4. Parenting which omits particular bonding modalities, and a responsive infant*

Amy (Case 3) exemplified this in failing to receive adequate holding. The mother was unable to perceive and respond to rising states of distress in her baby by holding her gently, close, and patiently.

*5. Parental overstimulation of the child*

This is exemplified by the family of Ken (Case 10) where the parents repeatedly overstimulated their son across several attachment and bonding modalities, but at the same time they did not assist him or allow him to make any sustained contact with them. Thus overstimulation is functionally allied to other interferences and omissions of attachment since it interrupts contact as readily as it establishes it.

---

**TABLE 9-2** *Specific patterns of disturbed behavior*

---

a. Infant lack of anticipatory posturing and molding with holding; lack of facial excitement in parents' presence; avoidance of eye-gaze with parents (Tony, Case 2; Bert, Case 7).

b. Maternal avoidance of eye-gaze with baby (Joan, Case 1).

c. Maternal avoidance of body contact and holding (Amy, Case 3).

d. Parental interference with touching, gazing, holding, and affective reciprocity with the baby through overstimulation of the child (Ken, Case 10).

e. Interference with the baby's attachment to one parent by the other parent: maternal overcontrol of and struggle for possession of the child (Edward, Case 4).

f. Interference with the baby's attachment due to maternal physical absence in the first year of life, and traumatic surrogate parenting (Jean, Case 9).

g. Inadequate support of bonding through maternal absence of involvement and lifelessness secondary to emotional unavailability (Ethan, Case 6).

h. Interference with attachment due to a feeding disturbance secondary to maternal depression and a baby's aggressiveness (from a case not reported in Chapter 6, but described in Massie, 1980).

i. A mother's aberrant avoidance of her baby in response to her cries of distress (Amy, Case 3).

---

184

Reported in Chapter 7, the ratings of parent-infant interaction empirically supported the relatively precise descriptions and categorizations of behavior which the individual case studies provided. Three judges, using a scale of mother-infant attachment indicators devised for the project, studied unedited films of the first six months of life of prepsychotic and control group families. Uninformed as to which group the films came from, the judges rated each scene of mother-infant interaction appearing in the movies. They found that mothers of infants who became ill appeared to touch their babies less or withdraw more from their babies' touches than control group mothers. The same appeared true for eye gazing—there was less initiation of and more avoidance of gazing among index group parents. In these modalities the infants in the two groups appeared indistinguishable. Both mothers and infants in the prepsychotic group seemed to mold, cling, and hold with more avoidance, stiffness, and less responsiveness than their control counterparts. When feeding scenes were observed, there were no differences in parent-infant behavior in the two groups.

*The Appearance of the Earliest Signs and Symptoms of Childhood Psychosis*  Reviewing Table 6-1 at the end of Chapter 6 reinforces the finding that most of the specific symptoms of early childhood psychosis occurred in our cases between six and twelve months of age, with a clustering between nine and twelve months.

**TABLE 9-3**  *First symptoms of psychosis, typically between six and twelve months*

Seeming hallucinatory excitement.
Appearance of self-absorption.
No visual pursuit of people.
Looking away from people repeatedly.
Avoiding mother's gaze.
Resisting being held; arching torso away from parents.
Autisms: hand-flapping, finger-dancing movements, rocking.
Plastic expressions: fleeting, unstructured, not communicating affect or intention; labile shifts from grimaces to squints.
Fragmented, uncoordinated body movements.
Episodes of flailing, aimless, unmodulated hyperactivity.

All of the children suffering from autism or Mixed Form of Early Childhood Psychosis showed one or more of these symptoms during the second half of the first year. By contrast, the two children suffering Symbiotic Psychosis of Childhood did not have these or any other observable symptom during this period. Amy (Case 3) showed a flattening of affect at fifteen months; and Edward (Case 4) did not appear ill until his third year. Then he, like Amy, became severely regressed when separated from his mother for nursery school. This relatively distinct profile for the children suffering Symbiotic Psychosis of Childhood supports the view that it is a different syndrome from autism and Mixed Form of Early Childhood Psychosis.

Major symptoms of firmly entrenched and psychologically disabling disease were present in eight of the ten cases studied intensively in Chapter 6 in the second year. The exceptions were Edward (Case 4)—one of the children suffering the symbiotic illness that became apparent only in the third year—and Bert (Case 7), suffering Mixed Form of Early Childhood Psychosis, who still only suffered the initial symptoms he had first shown between nine and twelve months.

**TABLE 9-4**   *Symptoms of established illness typically in the second year*

Child doesn't approach parents.
Keeps distance from parents.
Constricted or flattened affect.
Little or no purposeful activity.

In the film study what appeared most frequently in the *first six months* of life are *signs* of unusual development. Signs, however, are not *symptoms* of illness, since the same behaviors are seen in many normal children for days and even months in very early life. In healthy babies they pass with time and seem to bear little if any relationship to the normal child's later development. Only the specific motor deviations that we observed in Bert (Case 7, Mixed Form of Early Childhood Psychosis) are traceable directly to organic neuromuscular damage. In infants who develop normally, the remainder of the signs—typified by such qualities as flaccidity or irritability—may derive from constitutional differences, maturational imbalances, and also specific but transient adaptations to the caretaker. Nonetheless, one or more of these early signs were far more frequent and pronounced in the films of all of the children who subsequently acquired an early childhood psychosis compared to the films of normal infants. Thus it is likely that they mark the first steps in the process of illness that was to compromise severely the psychological growth of the group of afflicted children. In general, the babies' unusual behavior in the first six months of life is less involvement and pleasure with people and things in their environment than typical infants demonstrate.

**TABLE 9-5**  *Signs of unusual development in the first six months of life*

Flaccid body tone.
Lack of attentiveness or response to people or things.
Lack of excitment in presence of parents.
Lack of anticipatory posturing on being picked up.
Vacant, unfocused gaze.
Less than normal activity, such as reaching.
Specific motor deviations, i.e., developmental head lag on being pulled to sitting, submental palsy, ptosis.
Absence of molding to mother's body.
Eye-squint mannerism.
Predominantly irritable mood; little smiling.
More somnolent than typical child.

*Early Cognitive Development in the Disturbed Children*  There were films of fourteen children available for the study of intellectual development in the first years of life. To recapitulate the principal findings reported in Chapter 8, the children suffering an early childhood psychosis showed three patterns of stunting of cognitive maturation: *Group 1 were slowed* but nonetheless showed progression through Piaget's six sensorimotor stages to the point of understanding cause and effect relationships, acting with intention, and gaining the capacity for object permanence. In this category was an autistic child with moderate relatedness, a child suffering Symbiotic Psychosis of Childhood (Case 3, Amy, and a child with Mixed Form of Early Childhood Psychosis. *Group 2 were arrested* in cognitive development, showing some limited capacity for appreciating cause and effect relationships and acting on objects for the purpose of goal-directed behavior (sensorimotor stage 4). In Group 2 were four autistic children, a child diagnosed as a Symbiotic Psychosis of Childhood, and one suffering Mixed Form of Early Childhood Psychosis. *Group 3 were primitively fixated* at the lowest level of cognition in the first three years of life. At this level, body-centered actions predominated, and there was little sense of distinction between the self and objects in the outside world. Three of these children were autistic (Steven, Jean, and Ken—Cases 8, 9, 10 in Chapter 6) and one suffered Mixed Form of Early Childhood Psychosis (Ethan, Case 6).

It became apparent that the autistic children in our series were more likely to have the more severe interferences with cognition than the children with other forms of early childhood psychosis. This is congruent with their greater impairment in interpersonal relatedness. In addition, when compared to controls, the children with one of the psychotic syndromes were significantly less active with inanimate and animate objects in their environment. Again the autistic infants were the least exploratory, manipulative, and inventive with objects.

## Psychological Formulations

*Intrapsychic Determinants of the Disturbed Behavior in the Parents*    We turn now to the internal conflicts, impulses, and fears that underlay the configurations of bonding that we observed on film. These could be reconstructed from first-hand treatment and clinical interviews with the children and their parents, and from studying case records and therapists' notes. What emerged was a series of important concomitants of disturbed behavior in our group of cases. In some families there was a core psychological conflict, and in others many emotional currents were operating at cross purposes with healthy development. The parental conflicts, impulses, and fears appear in Table 9-6 which pulls together the intrapsychic factors. As the table shows, sometimes a particular conflict could flow in several directions, causing diverse behavioral outcomes. And sometimes different conflicts in a parent or in different parents led to similar behaviors toward the children. They were generally unconscious, and they were awesome in their magnitude and power to disrupt behavior, which is what distinguished them from their existence in normal or less disturbed parents who frequently struggle with similar feelings.

---

**TABLE 9-6    *Parental intrapsychic determinants of disturbed actions***

---

1. Ambivalence about the child, paralyzing the mother in her actions with the baby.
    a. Ambivalence derived from identifying the child with hostile images of the grandparents, siblings, spouse, etc. of the parent.
2. Ambivalence about the maternal or paternal role, stemming from hostile identifications with grandparents, or from rejection of grandparents.
3. Overt hostility toward the baby, sometimes because of the sex of the child, expressed in sadistic behavior.

**TABLE 9-6** *Parental intrapsychic determinants of disturbed actions* (continued)

4. A need for parental dominance expressed in overcontrol of the child, and sometimes sadistic actions.

5. Disavowals of consciously or unconsciously experienced hostility or ambivalence expressed through reaction formations such as
    a. Overgratification of the child
    b. Extreme passivity with the baby
    c. Withdrawal or separation from the baby
    d. Inability to separate from the child.

6. Maternal perplexity, ignorance, or confusion about child care.

7. A parental feeling of personal inadequacy leading to use of the child as a public or personal confirmation of self-worth, often expressed through prematurely pushing the baby toward developmental milestones and independence.

8. Paranoid fears of being hurt, used, or depleted by the child, leading to rejecting or avoidant behavior or reaction formations against avoidance.

9. Maternal sense of helplessness, and submission to authority or dominant figures with surrendering of the child to the traumatic, often sadistic actions of such surrogate caretakers.

10. Parental depression draining the capacity for lively and timely response to the baby.

11. Parental narcissistic self-involvement, leading to insensitivity to the baby in the form of missing the baby's cues or personalizing the baby's behavior so that signals are misinterpreted. For example, the mother reacts to the baby's cry as a sign that the child dislikes her rather than a sign of the child's distress.

12. Parental preoccupation with marital strife rather than with the baby.

13. Maternal conflicts over voyeurism and exhibitionism leading to avoidance of looking at the baby or being seen by the baby, with ultimate difficulty in eye contact with the child.

14. Unusually compulsive needs in a parent to arrange, organize, clean, or control a child which take precedence over affective contact and spontaneous response, enjoyment, or play with the baby.

15. Child care which is characterized by severe anxiety on the part of the parents, which may stem from any of the determinants listed above.

---

The table highlights the intrapsychic data but does not adequately convey the nuances of emotions, defensive attempts, and surrenders to fears and impulses that characterized the families in the study. At least one family suffered each of the troubling problems identified above; however, the same internal forces were usually active in several families, although perhaps not equally powerfully. To explicate each of these findings and their close connection to the parents' external behaviors and potential connection to the developmental failures in the children would be to rewrite Chapter 6, which is not the intention

*189*

of this review. However, some discussion of the liaison between levels of data does help.

For example, ambivalence and hostility seemed especially to explain the unusual affectionate stimulation and gaze avoidance of Joan's mother (Case 1). She cared a great deal for her child and lovingly wished to turn the difficult girlhood she had passively endured into a joyous childhood for her daughter, which she could then vicariously experience. This accounted for much of her nurturing actions, but unconsciously her anger, if not paranoia, over mistreatment by her parents and her subsequent paranoia about authority figures in general led her to undo or cancel out her affection for her baby. Thus she initiated and inhibited pleasurable and fulfilling climaxes with the baby in sequences of actions lasting just seconds at a time. Eye gaze was prominent because it was so latent with meaning, emotion, and anxiety for the mother. To meet the baby's gaze might be to reveal her rage; but it also carried the risk for her that she might lose control of her ability to say "no" to the child (the nay-saying aspect of her ambivalence) and succumb totally to her affection for the baby. Such apprehension also bespeaks an anxiety over loss of ego boundaries and fear of fusion with the child.

Amy (Case 3) highlights the crippling effects on maternal function of a sense of inadequacy which in its uncompensated form can lead to perplexity, confusion, and distance from the infant. Although very caring for her baby daughter, the mother could not easily bring her close for fear she might harm her with the evilness she felt she carried inside, a misconception that her husband and mother-in-law only promulgated. At other times, trying to undo the guilt she felt over her distance and sense of badness, she could not relinquish the baby, thus impairing separation and individuation, and fostering a symbiotic condition.

For both of these girls—and for the other children whose parents were the victims of their severe neuroses and character disorders—infancy must have been experienced as often contradictory, tense without the predictable prospect of relief, chaotic without the gradual emergence of a sense of the shape of oneself and the world, and rarely joyfully novel.

*The Infants' Intrapsychic Experience*   Although our data comes from several sectors, when we try to piece together how babies think and feel we are on very shaky ground. We speculate deductively from observations of infants and reconstructively from the symbolic and actual meaning of words and play of somewhat older children who have achieved this level of sophistication. Nonetheless, even very young speakers are unable to recall what it felt like in infancy—during their preverbal two years when ideas and emotional states did not have the coherence that language later gives them. With psychotically disturbed youngsters, the problem is even greater since communication, if it does arrive, is very fragmented. Theoretically, we have been tempted by the idea that the dreams of older children and adults may correspond to the older baby's and toddler's awake experience of the world. That is, the baby thinks like the dreamer: events are telescoped and rearranged in time; contradictions and opposite wishes can exist side by side; single people and objects represent many people and things, and vice versa. This is the effect of the phenomena of condensation, displacement, and symbolism which characterize dream experience. In dreams, repressed emotions are often relived fully and intensely rather than partially, and, by contrast, people or objects often appear as fragments of their whole selves. Along with the possibility that dreaming corresponds to the older baby's and toddler's thinking, the reality experience of the psychotic child between three and six years—filled with so many of the distortions seen in dreams—may also recreate the mind of the normal preverbal child. In fact, as different aspects of the Early Natural History of Childhood Psychosis Study suggest, illness for some of these children seems to be a fixation or arrest at the most primitive stages of psychological development.

Aside from clinical deduction and induction, what concrete information does the project provide to assist us in conceptualizing the intrapsychic life of children suffering one of the early childhood psychoses? The case studies in Chapter 6 repeatedly show youngsters with fears of objects and people which bear little or no relationship to the actuality of the thing feared. Thus the terrors must represent displacement of fear onto a person or thing from somewhere else, or a fragmentation of the reality and a response to only an aspect of the whole. Our children show far more frequent and more pernicious projections onto their environment of internal states than normal children. For some of the ill kids, projections of anger merged into delusions of their own omnipotence or paranoid fears of retaliation that were beyond the control of their reality testing. The frequency and intensity of projections also bespeak the extreme instability of the psychological boundary of the self in relation to the other. This ego boundary fragility in turn helps explain a sense of vulnerability of the self and the intense fear of annihilation of the self in the face of even benign threats. For these children, internal dissolution in the form of panic must be commonplace, and so must be a self-preservation rage to abort impending dissolution.

The case histories and psychotherapies illustrated how rage was more frequent in the disturbed children, and affection rare or inconsistent. By contrast, autoerotic behavior was prevalent, with many of the babies often unusually self-absorbed and engaged in rhythmic and self-stimulating activities.

Several of the earliest symptoms that appeared on film are behavioral referents of this theoretical construction of the internal life of the prepsychotic and psychotic babies. For example, there are the symptoms of self-absorption, seeming hallucinatory excitement, and the autistic stereotypies. The signs of poor molding, irritability and somberness, and the symptom of avoidance all support a picture of the pain with which the baby experiences his environment. And the symptoms of aimless, flailing, purposeless activity, and plastic, labile, noncommunicating expressions indicate how the child must derive little meaning or order for himself in connection with his environment, at a time when other toddlers are rapidly discovering and integrating interconnectedness.

Finally, the assessment of cognitive function using sensorimotor development pins down how little capable the psychotic and prepsychotic young children are to even think, let alone feel and express; and further helps explain the lack of structuring and stability of ego boundaries in the disturbed children. In specific, they are unable to think how two or more actions become interrelated or lead one to the other; how objects and people have properties and qualities that may be used to achieve a goal or be depended upon; how the self may act with intention to make a desired result happen; and how objects and people may exist, even if they are not present, and may be mentally evoked by using one thing to represent another symbolically.

### Historical and Ancillary Information

*Later Course of Early Childhood Psychosis*    Although the attention of this study has been on the earliest history of the syndromes of psychosis, it would be an oversight not to look at the later lives of the children. The case studies in Chapter 6 also tell what the Project learned of the years after childhood. In addition, information is available for six additional children studied in other parts of the Project. The outcome for all of these children, however, is not the natural history of illness, since all of the children eventually received treatment, though of widely different kinds. By contrast, the findings of the first three years of life reflect the early natural history of the syndromes because intervention was minimal, if it existed at all during this time. Autism remained the primary diagnosis of all the autistic children in the project as they grew into later childhood, with the exception of Steven (Case 8). At ten years of age, he was reported to be having auditory hallucinations, and by that time a diagnosis of childhood schizophrenia would also be accurate. Still the autistic children showed considerable variation as their lives progressed. There were those who had been institutionalized and remained severely arrested in virtually all areas of their development, including speech. Others, such as Tony (Case 2) and Ken (Case 10), who had shown an initial arrest of sensorimotor cognitive development in the first three years of his life, were doing acceptable work in normal high schools and were eager to take normative steps toward independence. The residue of their autism was in their aloofness, tense rigidity, and concreteness, which were considerably more pronounced than that of obsessional neurotics.

The two children diagnosed as Symbiotic Psychosis of Childhood (Edward, Case 4; Amy, Case 3) have remained seriously impaired— less well off than the autistic children with the better outcomes. Now in later childhood, both children require intensive daytime therapeutic support and show little ability to socialize with peers. With relatively well-developed speech, Amy has voiced delusions and Edward has communicated hallucinations. Although both children remain closely tied to and dependent on their mothers, at this time in their lives a diagnosis of childhood schizophrenia is also consistent with their symptomatology.

The four remaining children had been diagnosed as Mixed Form of Early Childhood Psychosis, and indeed they remained this way as they grew older, defying more specific labels by their highly variable pictures. The children, in their later childhood, have considerable speech, and they have periods of much affection for peers and their parents. They do show a push to separate from their families, yet they remain quite ill. They are often very awkward, concrete, prone to rage reactions, rigid, sometimes bizarrely manneristic when stressed, and often extremely anxious about new experiences. Their intense fears suggest possible delusions, but this is not a clearly developed symptom in any of the children. Cases S.H. and C.H. are especially interesting because of certain clinical correspondences. They were the two children who appeared "motorically driven" from the first weeks of life and never molded to their parents, and their outcome has been in one major respect different from that of all of the other children. As they grew older, they became increasingly aggressive and destructively impulsive. C.H., in adolescence, once used his considerable intelligence to fashion an explosive device which he placed in his psychiatrist's office. This tendency to violence in both children raises the question of a paranoid process or unsocialized aggressive (sociopathic) syndrome.

*Medical History*   Of sixteen children whose infancy films were studied closely in one or more aspects of the project, nine had organic medical findings. These were Robert (Case 5)—threatened miscarriage, mild toxemia, twinship; Ethan (Case 6)—intermittent slight bleeding during gestation; Bert (Case 7)—paralysis or absence of the right depressor anguli oris muscle; Steven (Case 8)—flu-like illness in the second trimester, headache, and edema; Jean (Case 9)—slight bleeding in the first trimester; S.I.—three previous miscarriages, heavy spotting first trimester; F.D.—threatened toxemia third trimester; C.H.—mother older than forty, with history of several previous miscarriages; Q.E.—hyperemesis second trimester.

## Conclusion

Having reviewed findings from all aspects of the project, it is tempting to look for groupings and then correlations among them. Yet we resist this because correlations between classes of findings such as, for example, diagnosis and medical history in such a relatively few cases would not achieve statistical significance. In addition, it is extremely hard to know how to integrate information arrived at with such varying methodologic approaches. There is the relatively "hard" descriptive data of symptom identification and cognitive staging, the more qualitative, though still statistically significant, assessment of bonding variations in parent and child, and the inferential clinical construction of parent and child intrapsychic phenomena. Nonetheless, we shall essay a few groupings and relationships here to build upon in the next chapter.

First, we termed several infants "unresponsive" (Tony, Case 2; Steven, Case 8; S.I.) because they appeared extremely passive and flaccid in the first month of life to a greater degree more than that observed in other children with these qualities. And two children were categorized as "motorically driven" (S.H. and C.H.) because from birth they were constantly restless and obviously difficult to console and hold. These qualities of extreme unresponsiveness in some children and motor driven-ness in others may very well reflect an underlying organic diathesis toward illness, but it is by no means certain that it could not also be a constitutional variation or the result of adverse or troubled caretaking in the first days or weeks of life.

Another breakdown of our findings which seemed potentially informative was to group prepsychotic children according to the kind of parenting they had received. "Traumatic parenting" was child-care where we observed the parents making distinctly dangerous "errors of commission," such as pushing a child away or not allowing eye contact to occur. This group included Joan (Case 1), Edward (Case 4), Amy (Case 3), Robert (Case 5), and Ken (Case 10). We also included Jean (Case 9) in this group because of her several-month separation from her mother in her first year. "Inadequate parenting" was mothering characterized by "errors of omission," such as a mother's not molding to a child or passively observing a child's fretfulness without alleviating its distress. Children experiencing this kind of care were Tony (Case 2), Ethan (Case 6), and Steven (Case 8) from Chapter 6, and Cases S.I., S.Q., F.D., and Q.E. discussed in other phases of the investigation. Only two cases (Bert, Case 7; C.H.) received "unremarkable parenting," a phrase which means that their mothering was indistinguishable from that observed in typical movies of control families.

One clear relationship appears here: only two of seven children who experienced what we described as traumatic parenting had a medical history of perinatal or gestational organic problems, while seven of nine children with parenting omissions (inadequate parenting) or unremarkable parenting had positive medical findings. This trend supports the case study findings which suggest that certain discrete kinds of severely traumatic environmental experiences can cause a psychotic syndrome in and of themselves. On the other hand, where parenting is either adequate or faulty by omissions of responsiveness, it is likely that there is a contributing organic factor when psychosis eventuates. Similarly, there is a slight trend toward a higher incidence of medical findings in the children whose cognition was arrested in the first three years of life (six of eight children) as com-

TABLE 9-7  Summary of major findings from different phases of the early natural history of childhood psychosis project

| | 1 Joan | 2 Tony | 3 Amy | 4 Edward | 5 Robert | 6 Ethan | 7 Bert | 8 Steven | 9 Jean | 10 Ken | 11 S.I. | 12 S.Q. | 13 S.H. | 14 F.D. | 15 C.H. | 16 Q.E. |
|---|---|---|---|---|---|---|---|---|---|---|---|---|---|---|---|---|
| **Diagnosis** — Autism | ✓ | ✓ | | | ✓ | | | ✓ | | ✓ | ✓ | ✓ | | ✓ | | ✓ |
| Mixed Form of Early Childhood Psychosis | | | | | | | ✓ | | | | | | ✓ | | ✓ | |
| Symbiotic Psychosis of Childhood | | | ✓ | ✓ | | ✓ | | | ✓ | | | | | | | |
| **First 12 months movie observation** — Traumatic parenting | ✓ | | | | | | | | | | | | | | | |
| Inadequate parenting | | ✓ | ✓ | ✓ | | | | | | | | | | | | |
| Unremarkable parenting | | | | | ✓ | ✓ | | ✓ | ✓ | ✓ | ✓ | | ✓ | ✓ | | ✓ |
| Unresponsive infant | | | | | | | ✓ | | | | | | | | ✓ | |
| Motorically driven infant | | ✓ | | | | | | ✓ | | | ✓ | | | | | |
| Medical history of perinatal or gestational physical problem | | | | | ✓ | ✓ | ✓ | ✓ | ✓ | ✓ | | ✓ | ✓ | ✓ | ✓ | |
| **Sensorimotor intelligence in first 3 years** — Cognition arrested or regressed | ✓ | | | | ✓ | ✓ | | ✓ | ✓ | | | ✓ | | ✓ | ✓ | |
| Cognition progresses | | | ✓ | ✓ | | | | | | ✓ | ✓ | ✓ | ✓ | ✓ | ✓ | ✓ |

pared to children who showed intellectual progression (two of six of these babies had medical findings).

Table 9-7 brings together for review several of the different classes of findings recapitulated in this chapter.

The next chapter synthesizes the many strands and levels of the project. In so doing, the investigation builds an etiologic model for early childhood psychosis. It also augments our model of normal psychic structuralization in the infant from the building blocks of mother-infant interaction and parental psychology.

# Chapter 10

# Synthesis into an Etiological Theory of Psychotic Development

Following our metaphor of navigating a swamp, here our currents begin to come together. Project data and understanding built up gradually from many sources converge so that we can map the onset of childhood psychosis in a significantly more precise fashion than has heretofore been possible. First there are the outlines of the map. These provide the same lay of the land which investigators and clinicians have charted for some time, but it is an etiologic schema worth presenting as a point of reference before proceeding into new territory.

The hypothetical model in Figure 10-1 is like a railroad switching yard in its multiple possibilities. For example, a healthy newborn may bypass the morass entirely and continue into a healthy childhood. Similarly but unfortunately, a child born with a genetic predisposition to psychosis (a genetic factor postulated to exist, but as yet unconfirmed) may also bypass intervening variables and continue on a straight line to profound illness. Yet for many children the passage through infancy is more tortuous. Thus, according to our model, healthy infants may experience traumatic parenting or other external

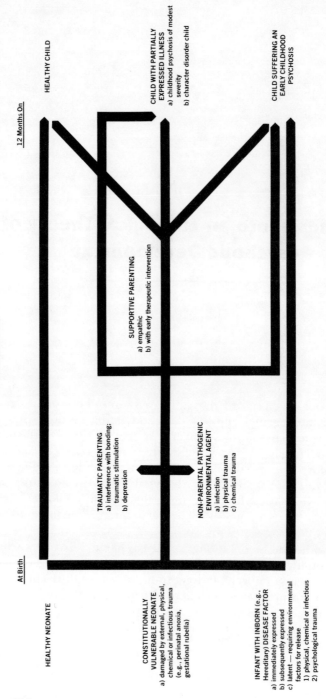

Figure 10.1   Etiologic model of early childhood psychosis.

insults, and, with or without therapeutic intervention, they may go on to develop illness of varying degrees of severity; they may also over-come and make healthy adaptations to life. Also of especial interest are the pathways by which physically vulnerable children and chil-dren with hypothetically inherited disease grow. They may escape syndromes of childhood psychosis altogether under optimum circum-stances if they avoid exposure to what are called "releasing agents"— psychological trauma and physical, infectious, or chemical noxious factors in their environment that perturb normal growth.

The possibilities in this switching yard are many, and the Early Natural History of Childhood Psychosis Project has focused especially on the section that involves psychological trauma which is related to disturbed parenting. Healthy, vulnerable, and genetically stigmatized newborns may all enter this domain. Then, in our studies, we have tried to understand what happens to the developing psyche of these children when the interaction with the parent is not normal. If the child's capacities are intact, the disturbed parent builds and fuels an abnormal relationship; if the child is born stigmatized or impaired, this too contributes to an abnormal dyadic process with the parent which becomes internalized and effects the evolution of the child's representations of the self and others.

In this chapter we want to reexamine our research findings against the background of the basic phenomenology of normal infant devel-opment put forth in Chapters 3 and 4 in order to delineate how the baby, in concert with impaired parenting, may create an aberrant psychological process that eventuates in early childhood psychosis. The data from the ill children and from normalcy fall into four major areas:

1. Gaze behavior. This was disturbed in several of our research cases. It is also central to mother-infant attachment, to discrimination of the self from the other, to the psychological process of internaliza-tion, and to overall psychic structure formation.

2. The use and balance of distal and proximal modes of caretaker-infant interaction—mother and child touching, vocalizing, gazing, holding and clinging, and affective interchange. They seem particu-larly implicated in the childhood-psychosis families. They are also fundamental to the baby's early acquisition of affective and motor schema of the self in concert with the mother, and, later, in the baby's capacity for self-regulation of internal states and comprehension and communication of meanings, intention, and moods through language and age-appropriate facial expressions and gestures.

3. The evolution of psychotic mentation in infancy and how it is interconnected with 1 and 2.

4. The psychodynamic understanding of the appearance of primitive defensive behaviors, then primitive defenses and symptoms; their relationship to the abnormal interactional phenomena and psychotic mentation; and, finally, their evolution into psychosis.

## The Etiologic Significance of Aberrant Mother-Infant Gazing

As discussed in the review of normal development in Chapters 3 and 4, the very young infant has some capacity to follow visual stimuli, to discriminate among the various things it sees, and to form percepts of objects and of facial schema. In fact, vision is perhaps the most highly developed neuromuscular response system for the newborn. Thus vision deserves special consideration as the principal faculty that organizes the baby's sensory experience, and the mother is an important organizer of the infant's early visual life. The features of the human face are a stimulus and configuration that can focus and hold the baby's attention often more successfully than competing internal and external events. The baby's vision aids in building a specific attachment to the mother, a differential response first to the human face and later to the mother's, and a memory for external events and people. Thus vision in the infant with an intact sensorium—in a reciprocal relationship with both the animate and inanimate environments—facilitates social development and psychic representations. If the reciprocal relationship is disturbed, the complex process by which vision organizes perceptual experience and builds internal figurative experience becomes subtly derailed. There result disturbed mental representations of significant people, starting with the mother. Likewise, the baby's self-image, growing from the matrix of the mother-infant self-object, also becomes impaired.

What is the mother's role with her baby in the dyadic newborn-caretaker visual system? On the basis of naturalistic observation and the experimental evidence mustered in Chapter 3, we understand how the mother responds to the child's gaze toward her, draws the baby's interest to her face, perceives her child's facial distress, and offers her own sympathetic or happy smile in return. And we understand how the maternal actions entrain the baby into a relationship with her as first representative of the world and provide the infant with a first sense of order and mastery in being able to elicit a contingent response. Incorporating these events, the baby gains his first experience with order and anticipation. The ability to anticipate is inherent in the infant's nascent though transitory self-regulation of internal distress. This affords the child its first experience with self-modulation of affective states, principally anxiety, for when a child can anticipate the sequence of events, it "knows" whether the next moments will bring pleasure or discomfort. When gratification is foreseen, there need be less anxiety. Further, the state of being able to anticipate in itself provides the child a measure of pleasurable control.

By contrast, blind or premature infants may give their mothers less visual cueing than normal children, and they have been described as having "little sending power" (Philips, 1980). With these babies, Field (1981) found that the mothers had to be unusually active in providing visual cues in order for preterm infants to gaze at the maternal visage as much as full-term infants did. In general in infants, "gaze behavior differences appeared to be a function of the varying amount of stimulation provided by the interaction partner" (p. 309). Field also found that infants showed less gaze aversion with the moderately active parent than with the minimally active parent.

Thus visual behavior between mother and child is highly interactional, but what happens if a caretaker violates the baby's need or anticipation of a response of a certain configuration, intensity, or timing? The research of the Brazelton, Tronick, and Als groups experimentally addresses this through their simulation of violated infancy expectancies. Discussed in Chapter 3, they delineate a hierarchy of goals of early mother-infant social interactions—initiation, mutual orientation of the partners, greetings, exchange of affective information, and mutual disengagement. They state that "both participants reciprocally modify their actions based on the feedback they receive from the other partner" (Tronick et al., 1978, p. 2). This is demonstrated in their experiment when the mother violates any of the goals and implicit expectancies of the normal face-to-face situation. The mother greets her baby, first in her characteristic animated manner, then with a still (expressionless) face which violates the baby's visual anticipation of the mother's affect. The infants, younger than six months, attempt to evoke the usual pattern of interchange with their mother through grins, activity, and gaze. Then they become dysphoric (apparently anxious), shut down, and grow still, expressionless, and withdrawn for a brief time.

This brief review highlights the important principles inherent in mother-infant gaze. It builds to our finding in the Childhood Psychosis Project that there was an early problem in mother-infant gazing in several cases. It was especially evident in Case 1 (Joan) where the difficulty seemed to arise from the mother. Similarly Cases 4, 8, 10 also revealed parents' difficulties maintaining eye contact with their children or responding to their gaze. However, in these families mutual gaze was but one of several disordered interactional parameters. Further, in no sense was our film evidence sufficient to rule out the possibility that there may have existed in these children when newborn an even more subtle violation of infant initiation of gazing and response to the maternal visage. That is, an organic interference with neonatal visual activity may impair the capacity of an emotionally vulnerable mother to entrain her child into the cycles of gazing and thus into a relationship with her. Conversely, a vigorous and undaunted mother could theoretically overcome a physical liability in an infant. We have observed this in case studies where therapeutic support of a mother can lead her to defeat reticence, ambivalence, and inhibitions, and reestablish a normal relationship with a child showing early signs of autistic withdrawal. Different from the families in which the mothers were not forthcoming was Case 7 where the baby was apathetic and at times did not seem to fix his eyes on people or things. His mother, on the other hand, was attentive, whereas the father was physically aggressive and rejecting with the child and mother.

In these cases, the mothers often, and the newborn sometimes, withdrew from normal excitement promoting interaction. It was this excitement that Robson and Moss (1970) noted as typically present at about six weeks of age. The women they studied reported at this time a sense of intense love and the feeling that their babies were "more of a person" when the babies looked at them. These feelings had "something to do with being recognized in a highly personal way." What parents generally prize seemed unsettling, especially to Joan's mother (Case 1) who avoided looking at her infant as well as at people in general. Nonetheless, she did feel affection for her child, and her contradictory nurturing and frustrating of Joan was the referent of an internal conflict in the mother that ultimately seemed to contribute to a shut-down in the child's attempts at human contact. We gathered from our psychotherapeutic contacts with Joan's mother that her conflicts over eye gaze represented a fear of expressing her considerable aggression if she looked too strongly, and also a wish to love and be loved that was at times so intense that if her eyes met another's there was a risk to her of fusing with her child or the other person with a loss of ego boundaries and panic-provoking ego dissolution. Additionally, the surrendering up of herself in an affectionate gaze also contained the dangers of rendering herself defenseless against a rejection and losing her capacity for independent functioning.

In other Childhood Psychosis Project cases we repeatedly observed caretakers stimulating babies and then not meeting their look; or stimulating a child so frantically that the child was physically not able to meet their eyes; or greeting the baby's smiles with frowns or anger; or drawing the infant away from dyadic gaze with a parent or other person. Taken as a whole, the deviations from the normal pattern of mother-infant gazing implicate the phenomena in the ontogenesis of profound psychological disturbances whose roots are in infancy. The data suggest that disordered infant visual responsiveness and perception and/or disordered parental stimulation of and response to infant gazing may interfere with several of the basic mental structures posited to exist in the first few weeks of life which form the substrate for ongoing mental development. In this way, (1) the baby's capacity to recognize the array of visual stimuli that results from its own and its parents' behavior may suffer. (2) The infant's ability to build up visual schema and consequently to maintain a percept as familiar or discrepant against competing stimuli may suffer. This is the anlage of self-regulation of anxiety through the capacity to anticipate future events by comparing present experiences with past experiences. (3) The infant's capacity for selective attention or inattention may suffer in the face of under- or overstimulation. (4) A baby's ability to sense causal relationships between itself and its mother may falter in the course of aberrant dyadic gazing. Each of these elements are early way-stations in the process by which the child gains an early sense of itself and sense of self as separate from the other.

## The Etiologic Significance of Parent-Infant Social Interaction

Although visual interplay with the mother—especially incorporation of the mother's image—is a formative influence in psychological development, it is but one of several elements which comprise mother-infant interaction. We must look at how gazing, touching, vocalizing, holding and clinging, and affective interchange are all patterned. As we saw, the newborn has certain capacities for each of these activities which then release an innate response in the mother.

Similarly, the mother entrains the newborn into cycles of continuing social behavior. The way this unfolds in any given dyad is highly variable within the range of what is normal. For instance, touching and holding (and infant clinging) are proximal (i.e., close) modes of relating, while mother-infant gazing, vocalizing, and affect are distal forms of interchange emphasizing the communication and perception of signals at a distance, the one from the other. One parent may utilize distal modes far more than another, as well as significantly underplay certain behaviors. Similarly, there are cultural differences in such patterning. Western industrialized societies engage their infants far more through distal communication than non-Western cultures, which place greater emphasis on bodily contact through holding. Within the normal range, differences in these behaviors may exert subtle but distinct effects on the emerging personality of the child.

But what happens when parent-introduced variations in these bonding and attachment behaviors exceed the developmental tolerance of the baby? Our discussion of aberrant gazing provided an illustration of its potential consequence in the form of disturbed differentiation of self and object representations, and its contribution to compromised self-regulation of affective states, principally anxiety, through its effect on anticipation. In this manner our attention is drawn to the *patterning* of social interaction; the interplay of distal and proximal elements; their rhythm as expressed in the timing of initiation, termination, response, maintenance, and synchronicity; and the force by which they are exerted. The parents' role in this reflects their own physical capacities, cultural values, and their psychological capacity for empathy with the baby. And the overall patterning, just like gazing, is a major building-block of the emerging personality of the child.

Thus we can conceptualize how the earliest organization of mother-infant interaction across *all* of the parameters just outlined brings the first sense of meaning to the child. Meaning has a cognitive component and an emotional component. On the cognitive side, embedded in the first mother-infant interchanges is the baby's initial sense of how one event follows another; how the mother-infant self-object can cause one thing to happen as a consequence of another thing; how, as the first months pass and self-object differentiation progresses, the self can have an effect on the mother and vice versa; and finally, how time is organized through events that lead the one to another, endure, pass, and return. All of this unfolds in the first twelve months, accelerating rapidly after the child leaves the symbiotic stage at about six months and enters the differentiation phase (Mahler et al., 1957). On the affective side, embedded in the mother-infant interaction are the child's first experiences of contentment, pleasure, excitement, pain, discomfort, and anger. These feelings in the first year of life are most often linked to a physiological state (but sometimes to novelty, mastery, motion, physical punishment, boredom, and frustration); the mother's response to it; and the baby's own response to the mother's intercession. For example, pain and anger arise in a young child over hunger. The baby imagistically and experientially links the distress with the-mother-as-withholding-food-and-relief. But when the mother offers her breast or bottle to the hungry baby in concert with her comfortable bodily support, distress shifts to contentment in the interaction with the mother. Moments later, contentment may give way to pleasure and excitement in shared physical play if the parent initiates rocking, cooing, smiling, and even tickling games in a manner consistent with baby's readiness for the games—that is, if the caretaker correctly perceives the baby's physical strength, muscular control, state of alertness, and labile shifts from excitement to fatigue.

We gain this understanding of the sweeping significance of the patterning of the several modalities of mother-infant interaction for emotional growth from the kinds of ethological observations and experimental studies discussed in chapters 3 and 4. For example, recall that we have been shown how babies learn to perform increasingly complex tasks when they are given responses that are contingent upon their actions. Likewise, babies in a state of overstimulation can attend less. Further, recall Stern's (1971) delineation of how the mother's voice and face are important arousers for the infant which leads to turn-taking of events between mother and child. The verbal and facial behaviors have parameters that are describable in their intensity, duration, speed, form, complexity, and frequency. Further, infants can match the intensity of stimulation experienced in one sensory modality with the intensity of a stimulus received in another modality. They also show some self-synchrony, so that the force of movement of the baby's body matches the intensity of its cry. In this way, it is likely that infants match and integrate the intensity and quality of a mother's voice with her touching and holding movements. In sum, when the mother's behavior is synchronous with the infant's state of readiness and capacity for response, we saw that the earliest psychological structures in the baby are schema of these sensorimotor experience; and, as Gouin-Decarie (1965) has described, building on the work of Piaget, the mother is at the intersection of the greatest number of schema for the infant. She can be sucked, touched, tasted, smelled, grasped, held, and seen, all in the parameters that Stern has described above which mother and baby codetermine.

In this way, a sense of meaning in the shared experiences with the mother, and images of the mother condensed from affective states in the shared experiences with the mother in the first year became internalized into the child's psychic apparatus. The mother clarifies emotional and cognitive meaning through sharing and example, and through her function as the baby's auxilliary ego which modulates excessive stimulation, frustration, and hunger. The powerful influence of cognitive growth and emotional experience in the relationship with the caretaker impels the child toward the major psychological milestones of animate object constancy and self-object differentiation which are reasonably well consolidated between the second and third birthdays. A communicative and cognitive step in this maturation occurs between the seventh and ninth month when the baby discovers that it can share a state of mind such as an intention with another person, typically the mother (Bates, 1976; Bretherton, 1981). This "intersubjectivity" is indicated, for example, by the baby's pointing and grasping with a cry at an object that it wants, while looking back and forth at its mother. This signifies the baby's awareness that it has a particular mental state at the moment and feels that the mother can share and reciprocate this state. The child's purposeful communication of affect with verbalization and gesture is the framework for early language: there is a medium for communication, and the appreciation of two separate minds which can nonetheless interface (Stern, 1982).

A further cognitive landmark is at approximately sixteen months when the child gains object permanence with the consolidation of the ability to remember an object which is out of sight. Object constancy is more complex and relates to the toddler's capacity to have and evoke a memory that is endowed with the affective qualities of a person, typically the mother. This mental representation of important people firms up at about three years of age (Mahler, 1975). The process is epigenetic, one stage building to the next by means of the baby's physiological states and visual, tactual, and auditory sensorium; and through the parents' facilitation of these states and modalities in social interaction which builds first the parent-infant attachment and, subsequently, the child's differentiation from the self-object state, which qualitatively and quantitatively eclipses the rudimentary behavioral distinctions with which the neonate enters life. In this way the toddler gains an internal representation of the parent that it can endow with loving and angry feelings. With the achievement of object constancy, the toddler can function comfortably away from the mother because it can evoke her benign image with the sense that she is someplace and that it will see her again. Still, when upset or separated from the parent for long periods, object constancy undergoes regression. The child becomes anxious, depressed, mistrustful, excited, and angry. The separated child may lose some independent functions (e.g., restful sleep, toileting, play); however, the normally developing child will recover when stresses such as illness or separation are over.

By contrast to the interactional ontogenesis of normal psychic structuralization, critical disharmonies were apparent in parent-infant behavior in the families of the subsequently ill children in the Childhood Psychosis Project. We have described how mothers in index families engaged less with their babies in touching, holding, looking, and affective sharing. The autistic infants also initiated less or avoided more eye gaze with their mothers than normal infants, as well as prepsychotic infants of other syndromes; and prepsychotic infants in general showed much less pleasurable affect and responsiveness with their mothers than normal babies. Therefore, whatever the initial cause or causes of these discrepancies between normal and troubled families, the infant's psychological experience of the interaction with the mother—the aliment of psychic structuralization—was different where psychosis occurred. In trying to pin down the experiential differences for the babies, we consider principally the mother's actions with the child here as in the detailed case studies in Chapter 6 since the data from the film study pointed in that direction when the families were taken as a group. Still some parents' behavior with their infants was normal or was undistinguishable at our level of examination from caretaking seen in families where less severe disturbances arose in the children. Further, as we have said, more concrete information on studies of perception and responsiveness in prepsychotic infants prior to diagnosis may appear in the future that could draw our attention to the initially disorganizing effect on mother-infant experience of subtle abnormalities in a baby's actions. This would require of the parents an extra degree of sensitivity and responsiveness, a task with which some families are more emotionally able to cope. Therefore, even as this may occur, still another reason for at-

tending to the parents' behavior is that in instances of dyadic disturbances in infancy, it is the adults (the parents and their therapist
allies) who must take the lead in directing the dyadic interaction toward health.

Experientially, the infants in our study suffered in several critical
ways from the imbalances in their relationship with their parents. In
Case 1 (Joan) we have spoken of the paradoxical message the mother
delivered to the infant through nuzzling her face and then avoiding
the baby's eye gaze—a preverbal double-binding request to look and
not to look at the mother with which it was impossible for the baby to
comply. Similar relatively clear paradoxes occurred in other families.
For example, in the families of Amy (Case 3) and Ken (Case 10)
parents excited the children by smiling at them and physically
stimulating them, but then did not respond with gratifying physical
closeness. Thus another way to conceptualize the sensate life of the
babies is that their parents did not understand the *meaning* of the
babies' responses. The children received paradoxical communications. But equally important, they were misunderstood. Quiescence in
some of the children, for instance, frightened the parent into thinking that something was wrong, and led the parents to overstimulate
the baby (e.g., Case 10). Laughter in a child, for example, led some
parents to withdraw from their baby or to accentuate the excitement
beyond a child's tolerance (i.e., Case 8). In these families, the parents'
misunderstandings of the infants' intentions were chronic rather than
occasional—if we can ascribe intent to the combination of instinctual
urges, reflex responses, and desires a baby demonstrates.

The caretakers typically missed the meanings of the babies' actions.
The parents' cognitive difficulty in understanding when a child
wanted to look, be held, play or eat, for example, was linked to specific emotional conflicts in the adults as outlined in Chapter 4 and
reviewed for our cases in Chapter 9. Thus, a mother may be anxious
about the meaning or intent of a specific behavior in a child and avoid
seeing it. For example, a child's pleasure in playing and messing may
evoke in the parent—typically unconsciously—anxiety derived from
how they themselves were treated when small in these same activities.
This may lead the adult to deny, through repression, a child's need;
or to do to the baby what had been done to it through a process of
identification with the aggressor (A. Freud, 1966). In our series, such
parents physically and emotionally withdrew from their babies, or
punitively restrained them.

Experientially, the infants at risk in our series passed the first year of their lives being misunderstood because of the cognitive-emotional breakdown between them and their parents which was reflected in the dismutual interactions. This finding is consistent with the earlier studies of Wynne and Singer (1963) which demonstrated that families with a schizophrenic young adult or adolescent failed to communicate clearly or to understand each other's communications in a family ambience of isolation, anger, and depression. The investigators determined this through being able to match the Rorschach responses of parents and their ill progeny correctly to each other in a blind fashion when given the test protocols of a series of families. Nonetheless, since the children frequently had been ill for some time, it is possible that chaotic communication and distressing affects in the families were more effect than cause of the illness. However, our own case studies suggested that there were no *gross* disturbances of response to the mother during the first six months in all but one of the children reported in Chapter 6, and in all but two of the children in the larger series of twenty-five. Therefore, this kind of infancy finding supports Wynne and Singer's hypothesis that the phenomena of mutual misunderstandings—and the affective chaos, confusion, and perplexity it leads to—have a causative role in the onset of psychosis. It also supports other aspects of the theory of unconscious parental transmission of their pathological conflicts to children, a theory developed largely on the basis of reconstructions from older patients as described in Chapter 4.

For such phenomena to exert a major pathogenic influence on psychological development, they must not be isolated occurrences. Rather they would have to take place consistently throughout infancy. In fact, our case studies do suggest that interactional disturbances particular to each parent-infant dyad were part of the fabric of family life. Antecedents of the disturbed parental behavior appeared in some cases before the child was born, and the parents' interpersonal difficulties continued within the family long after the child's illness became established, as well as in the parents' modes of relating to nonfamily members.

Chronically missed meanings and paradoxical messages exert their toll on the infant through not providing the baby with developmentally critical contingent response; by not entraining the baby into dyadic parent-infant interaction; through confusing the child with discrepant responses; by overstimulating the baby; through inducing a state of bored understimulation; and by causing a state of heightened frustration and organismic tension. Relating these phenomena of aberrant parent-infant behavior to the earliest mental structures of the baby outlined in Chapter 4, we can see where damage is likely to occur. As with disordered parent-infant gazing, the baby's ability to discriminate stimuli that result from its own and its parents' behavior may suffer, as will its ability to create sensorimotor schema from the experiences with its parents and to maintain percepts as familiar. The infant's capacity for control of attention may also suffer in the face of incongruous stimulation, and it may lose the recognition of causal relationships between itself and the parents. In addition, we also anticipate that disordered patterning of parent-infant behavior will obscure the child's establishment of temporal relationships. There is also likely to ensue damage to the child's ability to perceive the intensity of stimulation; to recognize whether sensation comes from within or without; and to register sensation motorically itself with verbalizations, or psychophysiologically through the autonomic nervous system.

Further, the phenomena of missed meanings and discrepant and paradoxical parental responses exert their pathogenic influence in still another fashion which in some respects is of a higher order psychologically than the disruption of basic mental structures. We conceptualize this as the failure of the parent and child to achieve affective consummations with each other.

Failures of affective consummation are a consequence of the misunderstandings of the meanings of behavior, missed perceptions of mood, and disharmonies among the various distal and proximal bonding behaviors. Consummations are potentially of particular importance because they are shared moments between mother and baby of heightened pleasure, excitement, quiet contentment, and even anger. The concept suggests a corollary to sexual climaxes or consummations during intercourse between adult partners which have a powerful influence on maintaining a couple's intimate bond. In parent-infant dyads, affective consummations, though not genitally sexual, function similarly. In addition, their developmental effect may be in the area of helping the infant gain a self-object representation through experiencing intense shared emotions with the mother first, then introjecting these experiences. This may be similar to what Kohut (1971) has described as the "transmuting internalization" which builds the self; and what Kernberg (1976) has described as the coalescing of affect fragments into self and object representations. From the self-object matrix the child differentiates a personal identity in the second year. This is significantly defined (and emotionally informed) by the consummate moments of pleasure, excitement, and contentment shared with the mother which have provided the baby with a confirmation of its existence.

In contrast to the depiction of the normal ontogenesis of the self, in the families of the Childhood Psychosis Project we observed a pattern of recurring failures of affective consummation. Behaviorally these were the times, for instance, when children became happy with their parents who then quickly stepped aside so the happiness could not be shared, and the children felt sad or angry (e.g., Case 8); times when excited children were so overstimulated that pleasure became pain, and the parents did not notice the shift in the child's mood and responded neither to the child's happiness nor unhappiness (e.g., Case 10); or instances when parents turned away from an angry child, neither confirming its tantrum with their own irritation nor assisting it to modulate its anger (e.g., Case 8); and for a final example, families where moodiness and inhibition allowed little to-and-fro pleasure between caretaker and baby (e.g., Cases 2 and 6). Infants in families such as these were liable not to make the step to self-object differentiation. If some differentiation did occur, they were liable to develop a "false self" (Winnicott, 1965) that was based more on imitation of others' behavior and emotion rather than growing from mutual parent-child events endowed with shared affective states.

In some of the Project families, and in our broader clinical experience, we observed parents who habitually misperceived and did not effectively manage their baby's increasing distress. It exceeded the child's capacity for self-pacification and internal regulation. Wild anxiety took over the baby, who became completely disorganized with loud wailing cries and flailing arms and legs. In the most extreme situations this suggested an organismic disorganization and dissolution of the baby's rudimentary ego or self. After a time the children "shut down" and stopped signaling for a response since none had been forthcoming. Some became apathetic.

Finally, this discussion of the implications of disturbed parent-infant interactions leads to the concept of empathy. Defined as a person's capacity to project one's own consciousness imaginatively onto another being, parental empathy has long been felt to be essential in nurturing a child. However, empathy is not a willy-nilly projection of personal feelings onto another, but rather an accurate perception of the other person's state, coupled with the appreciation of how one would feel if in that state. This appreciation, projected onto the other, provides the conviction that one knows how the other person is feeling and can respond accordingly, even if the other person cannot adequately verbalize his or her condition. We use the word "state" advisedly because, as outlined in Chapter 3, infants have five major states—deep sleep, quiet light sleep, quiet alertness, active alertness, and crying. Parental empathy involves the accurate appreciation of the baby's state and the associated feeling, which allows the parents to intervene effectively with the child.

The Childhood Psychosis Project families, and broader clinical practice, frequently reveal parents unable to empathize with their children. This failure encompasses the aforementioned misunderstanding of the meaning and intention of babies' expressions, and the dyssynchronous actions which follow. Case studies show why in some instances parents cannot empathize; for example, empathizing with an infant's distress requires the ability to know suffering oneself. However, in instances of pathology a parent may have suffered so much that she represses conscious acknowledgment of distress. Alternatively, a parent may identify with an aggressor who has made her suffer formerly and strike out at the distressed baby. Conversely, to empathize with an infant's state of quiet alertness requires the parent to have the capacity for passive contentment. But some parents find this so unnerving that they are unable to play quietly with a young child. In our experience, when there are failures of empathy children are not able to enter into the intersubjective dialogues with their parents in the second half of the first year. And more basically, the children do not receive confirmation for state-specific feelings, which prevents these moods from being incorporated into ego states. Instead the ego and self-object is an incomplete or fragmented amalgam. As Kernberg has described from his work with severely disturbed adults, fragments of affect which go into building the self-object had not coalesced in their childhood (1976).

Nonetheless, in some instances it is likely that the infant's own signaling of affective need state and state of arousal is defective or weak. This increases the likelihood of empathic errors, and puts a much greater burden on the mother.

## The Evolution of Psychotic Mentation in Infancy

From the disturbances in dyadic gazing, perception of moods, and parent-infant response across modalities, pervasive developmental problems arise. Although we have been concentrating on feeling, pathology does not spare thinking. We saw in Chapter 8 how the growth of sensorimotor intelligence was slow, arrested, or primitively fixated in the first two years of life of ill children. The autistic youngsters in general were more severely afflicted than those suffering other forms of childhood psychosis. It seems likely that the mechanisms that disrupt mentation and those that interfere with emotional life are closely connected. For with respect to both cognition and affect, the two-year-old toddler's crowning achievements are the abilities to act with intention to produce a desired result and to maintain a mental image. The first well-established living image is the mother's. We have seen how the infant's panoply of interactions with the parents outlines the human image which is then shaded in with the feelings that attend those interactions. Similarly, the image of nonanimate things grows from the experience of sharing behaviors, if you will, with objects. The baby's perceptual and motor capacities bring it into contact with things which, unlike people, do not typically share in initiating interaction. But once in contact with an object, the baby comprehends it through sensory and motor experience with the object: its weight, smell, appearance, sound, feel, taste, movement, and its response to the baby's manipulations. Likewise, the baby thinks (learns) about itself through sensing its own possibilities with animate and inanimate objects. The typical vigor babies have in exploring objects and their environment indicates an innate drive toward mastery of the nonhuman world. And like the child's drive to attach to its mother, inanimate object relatedness can also suffer when the child is limited by physical disability or perceptual interferences. This impinges upon early mentation which is inextricably bound to the child's image of its interactions with things. But inanimate objects, unlike many of the parents in the Childhood Psychosis Project, cannot willfully (either consciously or unconsciously) withdraw, misunderstand, or be contradictory. Inanimate things simply have many properties for mastering.

Still, our research suggests that the process of mastery can be powerfully impeded when there are critical interferences occurring at the same time in the baby's relationship with the caretaker. For example, if the infant experiences unreliability, intense discomfort, and repetitive episodes of noncontingent responses with the caretaker, that is likely to have an impact on its readiness to interact with the nonhuman world. Rather than pleasurable anticipation of mastery, bewilderment may inhibit the growth of comprehension of the rules of events and properties of things.

Under such circumstances, there are different possibilities for the child. It may turn primarily to things, and engage in ritualistic, very simple, sometimes reflex manipulations with them which are noteworthy for their repetitiveness. In this way the child withdraws from the more complex world of human beings or objects which have shifting properties. This characterizes severe autistic behavior, and what we have termed a primitive cognitive fixation in Chapter 8. Or the baby's interest in objects may continue, but comprehension is slowed secondary to the apprehensions and uncertainty that are the emotional and cognitive matrix of the maternal-infant relationship in cases of disharmony and that the baby then brings to his contact with the nonhuman world. Transference of the emotional valence of a disturbed dyadic relationship to sensorimotor learning is a phenomenon to which Anthony (1975) and Greenspan (1979) have already drawn our attention. In our own cases we have termed it "cognitive slowing" if the child gradually, but more slowly than normal, constructs a permanent image of objects complete with their attributes and the child's own capacities with these attributes. Finally, it seems from our own series of cases that some children are able to avoid primitive cognitive fixation, but to grow only so far in their ability to understand objects and how to manipulate them. We have spoken of these toddlers as suffering a "cognitive arrest."

Scrutiny of the index group of children in their behavior with objects according to Piaget's categories of the growth of sensorimotor intelligence allowed a further delineation of their mentation. As discussed more fully in Chapter 8, at two years of age, when many of the children had been ill for some time and others were showing their first symptoms, their thoughts seemed to be focused on their own bodies for the most part or upon the task of establishing the relationship between their bodies and another person or object. This is the cognition of sensorimotor stages 2 to 4 which normal children have surpassed in the second year of life. Many of the ill toddlers have little indication of a coherent sense of a self that has an existence separate from other people and things and that can act with intention toward them. In other words, the psychotic and prepsychotic youngsters were usually arrested in an attempt to make sense of the most basic perceptions as well as cause-and-effect connections between things, and they were fixated in self-preoccupation with body movement and sensations.

We can see three possible explanations for this: one, the drive to mastery has been thwarted because experiences with people have been extremely perplexing and disruptive so that interest remains focused on the simplest and most predictable things which, for the traumatized child, are surer and more satisfying; and two, the child's ability to process perceptual and motoric experiences is organically impaired. The third possibility, that the baby has been deprived of significant amounts of sensory and human experience so as succumb to a deprivation syndrome marked by helpless apathy and autoerotic repetitive behaviors did not occur in our series of families.

In addition, unlike normal two-year-olds, the prepsychotic and psychotic children rarely showed signs of thinking about an object or person's functions and usefulness; novelty was not especially interesting, and there was little or no trial-and-error exploratory experimentation with people, space, objects, and their relationships. It also follows that, with the exception of two children, there was no sign that the toddlers used an image of either a person or an object to figure out an action; there was no sign of symbolic representation, and imitation of people had not appeared, nor had imaginative or pretend play. This is consistent with the failure of verbal language in most of the children, for there was little or no use of words to regulate interactions, express needs, explore and question, announce and inform, or pretend. These are all basic language functions and signs of the achievement of early object permanence, object constancy, and differentiation of the self into an I and another. Instead, we must infer that the thoughts of the most seriously afflicted toddlers are largely objectless and timeless. Inner experience is fused with outer experience. People and things do not have substance; without reason, they cause pain and pleasure, so that magicality stamps the child's thinking. The child is both the source of all sensations and thus omnipotent, and at the same time impotent to effect a change in whatever happens. Thinking and feeling this way, the toddler's self-image is chaotic, at once terribly defective and all powerful. The world is filled with parts of the self, things, and the parents that shift like a kaleidoscope of gratifying, painful, mysterious, simple, and dangerous ideas.

In sum, factors described above in the social-interactional realm and in the perceptual realm profoundly disturb the infant's elaboration of cognitive schema. Schema are disordered because it is likely that there are interferences with several of the basic mental structures of early life: the child's capacity to recognize and maintain an image of stimuli and their source; the child's ability to recognize the temporal relationship of events and perceptions; and the baby's capacity to perceive causal relationships between itself, its mother, and inanimate objects. This interference with cognition so early in life has an ever-broadening effect on the child's ensuing comprehension of reality and interpersonal relationships.

## The Psychodynamic Understanding of the Appearance of Defense Behaviors, Defenses, and Symptoms

The study of aberrant mother-infant gazing, other disturbed patterns of attachment and bonding, and cognitive failures has led to an understanding of problems in psychic structuralization in young children suffering one of the early childhood psychoses. The next section of this chapter follows the trail to a discussion of how psychological trauma and early defects manifest themselves in pathologic defenses and symptoms. There is a hierarchy of defenses and symptoms that is consistent with the child's developmental phase. In the first six months of life, when the child is largely functioning at a psychobiological level, responses to threats are physiologic and motoric. In the general sense, a defense is anything that opposes attack, violence, or injury. Internal danger may be inner-need states which become intolerable, leading to disorganization; external dangers may be in the form of threats in the animate or inanimate environment. And the basic early life reactions are in the direction of physiologic conservation and withdrawal and motor fight and flight. After six months, with beginning psychologic structuralization, responses to danger become psychological, and symptoms reflect mental conflict. And by five years of age, with resolution of the oedipal complex, there has been sufficient elaboration of the id, ego, and superego that the entire defensive process occurs normally unconsciously and intrapsychically: id impulses disorganize or push for expression; the ego senses danger and signals anxiety; and the ego or superego erects a defense to manage or ward off the expression of what is internally felt to be dangerous. Restated, it has been our experience that dyadic interactional problems and psychologic structural failures very early in life lead stepwise to defense behaviors, then to pathologic defenses, and next to symptoms.

"Defense behaviors" is a term Fraiberg first used (1981) to describe phenomena she had seen firsthand in deprived and traumatized babies enrolled in her Infant-Parent Project. Her observations were similar to what we saw in the infancy movies of several of the prepsychotic children. Defense behaviors are different from subsequently appearing psychologic defenses in that the former are physical actions the babies use to ward off and manage danger; the latter are more complex in that they involve also a mental operation to achieve self-protection against both external forces and internal impulses. To elaborate, Freud (1922) described defenses as mechanisms of the ego used in states of conflict. They are mobilized (1) by anxiety that may arise from internal excitement or instinctual tension; (2) by anxiety arising from real external dangers to the self; and (3) by anxiety from the superego (conscience). Thus defenses not only are self-protective, they also often are mechanisms of mastery and control of the self and the environment, and modes of normal adaptation. Psychopathology results from a failure of defenses, and also from the continued use of developmentally early (primitive) defenses beyond the age at which they are normally employed, or their inappropriate use when less powerful or more sophisticated defense mechanisms should suffice. The primitive defenses which belong to the oral phase of life in psychoanalytic theory (the first eighteen months) are introjection, projection, denial, and splitting. Developmentally higher defenses are reaction formation, isolation of affect, and undoing, which appear next in the anal phase (approximately eighteen to forty-two months); later appear regression, turning against the self, reversal, repression, and sublimation (A. Freud, 1937).

We are particularly concerned with the primitive defenses since they are the first to emerge and are closely linked to the prior defense behaviors. Additionally, severely disturbed children beyond the second year use them inordinately. These children often are arrested at or show a regression to these mechanisms, or they are extremely slowed in acquiring more advanced defense mechanisms. It is these very developmental imbalances of defenses that are often the symptoms in psychotic children.

### Defense Behaviors

The following signs that we observed in the childhood psychosis cases in the first year of life, especially the first six months, may be defense behaviors: excessive somnolence, flaccidity, inattention, a gaze which remains vacant and unfocused after the first weeks of life, apathy or lack of excitement and smiling after the first two months,

**Table 10-1** *Developmental sequence from defense behaviors to symptoms in the first two years of life*

| Defensive behaviors | Primitive defenses | Symptoms |
|---|---|---|
| Withdrawal to sleep (includes somnolence) | Introjection | Depression |
| | Projection | Irritability |
| Gaze aversion (includes inattention, blank gaze) | Denial | Aggression (anger) |
| Motility (includes moving away, avoiding holding, pushing the other way) | Splitting | Anxiety and panic |
| | Displacement (from one body function system to another) | Need for sameness |
| Protest and fight | | Hallucinations |
| Shut-down (of individual sensory and motor modalities) | De-differentiation | Delusions |
| | De-animation | Autisms (flailing, hand and finger dancing, twirling, rocking, posturing stereotypies) |
| | De-individuation | |
| Substitution (of one sensory and motor modality for another) | Transformation of affect (e.g., turning against the self; reversal from passive to active) | Self-mutilation |
| | | Plastic expressions (lability that doesn't communicate mood or meaning) |
| | Undoing | Impaired relationships (avoiding or clinging) |
| | Isolation of affect | Cognitive arrest or delay in object permanence |
| | | Little purposeful activity |
| | | Preoccupation with objects |
| | | Speech failure (echolalic, metaphoric, arrested, repressed) |
| | | Disturbed response to pain, heat, cold |
| | | Low frustration tolerance phobias |
| | | Ego boundary confusion (failure of self-object differentiation and achievement of self and object constancy) |

NOTE: Defense behaviors are normal if transitory in response to temporary conditions. Likewise, primitive defenses are a step in normal psychological structuralization between approximately 6–18 months. Pathology occurs with fixation at these mechanisms or later regression to them.

inactivity, a physical withdrawal from attachment manifest in not molding or clinging to the parents, active attempts at pushing away the parents with arms or legs, and avoidance of the parents through not meeting their gaze and turning away from them. In Chapters 6 and 9, these findings were discussed as early signs of disturbance, with the proviso that they often appeared in normal children transiently and did not persist to become fixed characteristics. Further, several of these signs, such as flaccidity or hypertonic body-thrusting avoidance, may not necessarily have a defensive function; rather, they may reflect defective organically mediated responses to essentially normal environmental stimulation.

Here, however, we want to emphasize the potential self-protective nature of these behaviors from the psychodynamic point of view. Thus the signs, which range from a muscular absence of tone to a highly active avoidance of contact, may be the baby's way to avoid the kinds of overstimulation and confusing stimulation delineated in the study of parent-infant interaction. Several of our signs correspond to Fraiberg's description of withdrawal, a more general and inclusive term, as a defense behavior or reaction (1980), which she derived from direct observation of infants at risk with disturbed parents. Several of our signs are consistent with Greenacre's description of "defense reactions" (1958), which included reduction of responsiveness to external stimulation and withdrawal into fatigue or sleep. Her findings were derived from psychoanalytic reconstructions of the infancy of disturbed adults during treatment. Lastly, Mahler, through direct developmental observations of children, has classified related phenomena as "maintenance behaviors" (1968). She has described in particular "de-animation" as withdrawal from reality.

Fraiberg, Greenacre, and Mahler each list additional protective operations, and we come to them shortly. However, they require the initial presence of psychic structuralization in the form of early ego and id differentiation, object relations, and defense mechanisms in the second six months of life. Thus we prefer to call them "primitive defenses" along with the aforementioned introjection, projection, denial, and splitting. To reiterate, for the earlier actions which do not require psychological mental operations, we reserve the term "defense behaviors."

In considering the range of findings that may represent defense behaviors, it is possible to classify them into seven kinds of relatively discrete reactions. Each helps the infant avoid danger or diminish the impact of pernicious stimuli through the function of particular sensory and motor modalities. They are withdrawal into sleep, gaze aversion, motility, freezing, protest and fight, shut-down of individual modalities, and substitution.

1. *Withdrawal into sleep.* This is a primitive defense reaction involving a total withdrawal of organismic function. It can also be a simple response to both normally or pathologically occurring conditions. For example, if visual stimulation is too intense, too discrepant, or even too uninteresting, the organism may withdraw into sleep. In laboratory studies of infant vision, it has been noted that infants sometimes fall asleep if the stimuli are too simple or repetitive. Although total, sleep is quantitatively and qualitatively different than the massive or global defense behaviors against threats to the existence of the infant itself.

2. *Gaze aversion.* The visual modality can be utilized defensively in a number of reactions. The complexity of the visual system of the infant increases the frequency and kinds of defense reactions available to the infant through this modality. One of the most easily observable visual defense reaction is simple gaze aversion by which the infant turns its eyes away from an inanimate object or human stimulus. However, there are more complex and subtle modes of gaze aversion. For example, based on Haith's finding discussed in Chapter 2, we know that the infant scans constantly when awake, even in the dark. The constantly scanning eyes appear to fixate on objects, and yet in reality they could be blankly staring and not registering the image of the object toward which the eyes are directed as a form of gaze avoidance. To assess whether the baby was disengaging from contact in this way, we would have to measure whether the baby was targeting an image—such as the mother's visage—on the foveal area of the retina. This is the area of the eye where the form or pattern image occurs in babies of four months or older, and this allows them to make distinctions in facial configurations.

Head-turning itself is another way in which the infant averts gaze, bringing into play motility in the service of defense. The degree of head-turning depends upon the development of the child's musculature as well as the intensity or need on the part of the baby to break gaze.

3. *Motility.* To use motility defensively, the infant requires development and control of musculature in order to push itself away, to push the other away, or to use forms of locomotion such as crawling or

toddling. Like withdrawal to sleep and gaze avoidance, the baby attempts to get away from the source of the dangerous or aversive stimulus, a form of primitive denial. Motility often serves to avoid tactile stimulation. A parent may overstimulate by holding the baby too close or too forcefully, resulting in the child's attempting to push the parent away, to push itself away, or to appear to flail about in attempts to loosen the hold. Further, Main et al. (1982) demonstrated through microanalyses of mothers and their infants that mothers may give subtle rejecting signals from a distance that are nonverbal; the babies respond by moving away or ignoring the mother's more overt attempts to engage the infant. These behaviors are not necessarily evident until videotapes are studied in slow motion.

4. *Freezing.* This describes varying levels of infant immobilization from extreme to partial. It may occur at times in situations of paradoxical or double-binding stimulation from which the infant cannot use motility to escape (e.g., in the Childhood Psychosis cases when a baby is both physically overstimulated and smiled at simultaneously, the baby may lose its expression and become still and apathetic). The child may also freeze with totally incapacitating immobility in response to physical trauma (Fraiberg, 1981).

5. *Protest and fight.* Recognition of this comes from ethology (Bowlby, 1968). It is a reaction to the danger of loss, separation, or deprivation. Like primitive reaction formations, the infant attempts to ward off depression and fear in the actual situation through the expression of aggression. Thus unbearable feelings or internal disorganization are reacted against with protest and/or fight. Warding off internal disorganization, a young infant may flail about, fighting off attempts of the mother to "contain" it through holding and other caretaking interventions.

6. *Shut-down of individual modalities.* This defense reaction may involve the shut-down of all or part of the function of any sensory or motor modality. For example, the infant may go in and out of states of drowsiness, and it may have temporary inhibitions in motor activity and not move, or in vocalization and curtail babbling. At the extreme, a baby may shut down digestion with diarrhea, rumination, and regurgitation leading to an arrest of growth. A parent's overstimulation or paradoxical stimulation may thwart the child's activity, which could cause the child to lose initiative in sensorimotor exploration. In terms of cognitive development, if the baby does not gain the sense, or loses the sense, that its actions have an effect in the world—as a conse-

quence of experiencing the world as chaotic or discrepant—it may shut down responsiveness in a vulnerable modality or in the specific area in which it has not been reacted to contingently by its caretakers.

7. *Substitution.* This describes the defense reaction in which the baby uses one sensory or motor modality to mitigate a threat associated with another sensory modality. For example, if a mother finds it difficult to sustain gaze with her baby and thwarts its attempts to initiate gaze, the intact infant may use touch to engage the mother. Or as observed in Case 4 of the Childhood Psychosis Project, when a mother was unable to initiate close holding in order to respond to her child's strong affects, the baby took the lead with touches and gazing.

### Primitive Defenses

Chronologically, after the period of defense behaviors—which are reactions to pernicious stimuli—the child becomes capable of managing some stimuli and the associated affective states with intrapsychic processes. At this point, beginning approximately in the second six months of life, the child has begun using primitive defenses, not simply behaviors and reflex avoidance reactions. These early defenses are listed in Table 10-1. To this lexicon Fraiberg has contributed an understanding of transformation of affect. This is a primitive form of reversal, or turning passive into active, which she observed in a mistreated eighteen-month-old who relinquished sadistic actions for masochistic (self-hurtful) behavior. In addition, withdrawal develops rapidly into what both Fraiberg and we have called "primitive denial": turning away and protest give way in the deprived, confused, or abused baby to a state of silent apathy or a failure to register traumatic experiences verbally or facially.

Greenacre, in her discussion of the "equivalents of defense mechanisms before the full assembling of the ego" (1958), adds displacement, wherein a child substitutes one body-functional system for another. For example, in a troubled child tensions from the patterning of toilet control, from control of feeding, or even from disharmonious mother-infant gazing or physical closeness may invade speech development, leading to an arrest in language. Likewise, earlier in life similar tensions may interfere with appetite, digestion, or possibly trigger psychosomatic responses such as allergic skin disorders.

Each of these primitive defenses requires an early degree of internal representation, one that begins to appear in the second six months of life, whereby one affective state or a representation may substitute for another. Similarly, Mahler includes in her classification of maintenance behaviors dedifferentiation, deindividuation, deritualization, fusion, defusion. Each of these primitive defense processes involve regression from a higher stage of psychological development. Defusion is a retreat from normal mother-infant symbiosis into Mahler's autistic stage where the infant makes little or no distinction between internal and external experiences. The other processes are retreats to mother-infant symbiosis from subsequent stages of separation and individuation where some degree of advanced self and other representation had been achieved. Retreat from development occurs because anger and frustration, and the threat of physical separation from the mother threaten the child's sense of self. This arises where there have been the kinds of nonempathic interactions, which have not supported development, that we have been describing in the childhood psychosis families.

In Chapter 4 we described splitting as a normal but primitive process intrinsic to the first two years, in which the gratifying and frustrating maternal object becomes incorporated as the nucleus of the self-object. It subsequently is unified into one maternal representation during self and object differentiation. Pathological splitting may speak to an arrest of this process, so that in severe disorders, such as borderline states or psychosis, the object remains invested with irreconcilably ambivalent love and hate. It is also a primitive regressive defense whereby the individual protects the loved object from either obliteration of the mental representation or real destruction by splitting off the good image from the hated one. Again, consideration of the avoidances and nonempathic, discrepant interactions between mother and infant in the childhood psychosis families—experiences which heighten but do not resolve feeling—suggests that these are the behavioral substrate for the fragmented self and other images which splitting describes.

Additionally, as primitive defenses, introjection and projection deserve elaboration. Greenacre (1958) discusses how fundamental incorporate drives are vision, orality, and touch. Although her terminology is different, the phenomena she describes are analogous in some respects to what we earlier described in Chapters 3 and 4 as the schema building that evolves out of the baby's sensorimotor interactions with the mother. By these means the relationship with the mother "out there" is replaced by one with an imagined inside object;

and her mental representation continues her functions, but now in the infant's fantasy rather than reality. Emotions that the child has experienced in reality with the mother color the internalized object. As Greenacre points out, projection occurs when the infant's happy or distressing fantasies about the inner representation of the parent become too overwhelming. Thus if the child has felt great discomfort at the hands of the mother along lines we have described, the baby cannot feel pleasure or affection for the internal self-object representation. He rages at it, and when the destructive fantasies rise to the point of destroying the rudimentary self and other images, the rage is projected onto the environment. Through projection, the parent, strangers, or even inanimate objects become bearers of dangerous hostility. Further, chronic rage, whether inner directed or projected, renders the child's own self-image unlovable, defective, and incomplete. This further impairs maturation through its interference with the sense of competence and mastery that fuels the push toward self-object differentiation, libidinal object constancy, and individuation.

The projection mechanism is similar to the paranoid and depressive conditions Klein (1948) postulated in normal development in the first year of life. In brief, she described the infant's rage at being deprived of the breast (a real experience, as well as a metaphor for the inevitable instances when the caretaker cannot soothe the baby). The baby externalizes the rage onto the mother in what becomes a model for the attribution to outside forces of overwhelming feelings of helplessness and anger. We do not give this mechanism the primacy Klein does for normal development, however, seeing it more as a consequence of pathologically dismutual mother-infant dyads.

### Early Symptoms of Illness

In psychotic children, the path from disturbed attachment to the disturbed patterning of dyadic interactions, to defense behaviors, to interferences with psychic structuralization, to primitive defenses ultimately leads to symptoms of illness. Table 10-1 lists the major symptoms of the early childhood psychoses seen in the Project cases in relation to defense behaviors and primitive defenses. Prior discussion of some of these symptoms has demonstrated how they are mechanistically linked to earlier phenomena on the developmental ladder.

Other symptoms deserve explication. For example, *depression* in a general sense is a consequence of the child's loss of the mother. The loss may be real as Wolf and Spitz have described for anaclitic depression (1946) in the second six months of life, or it may be the loss of the internalized image of the mother and the contentment this image brings to the baby's self-image. For example, the case of S.I., an autistic child reported on in Chapter 8, suggests this. The child brightened at his mother's face and voice at five months, which indexed stage 3 sensorimotor cognitive function. He then lost this response to his mother, showing only stage 2 sensorimotor behaviors with inanimate objects until his third year of life. Because of dyadic and maturational failures, infants such as this one may never have adequately introjected the mother's image and the infant's aggression may destroy it. Symptoms of *infant clinging, panic at separation,* and the *need for sameness* are all likely to be connected with this same developmental disturbance in the baby's introjection of the parent and subsequent self-object differentiation and separation.

*Autistic stereotypies* and *self-mutilation* are symptoms which may help the ill baby establish a boundary for the self in the struggle to distinguish inner and outer experience when development has been fixated at this stage, or when, because of confusion at higher stages, the baby has regressed to this stage. Self-mutilation may also represent aggression turned against the self, utilizing the primitive defense of reversal or transformation of affect from the real outer-directed anger. It may also be an attempt to destroy a hated internalized object—to "cut out the offending part."

*Hallucinations, delusions, avoidance of people, preoccupation with objects,* and even *nonperception of pain, heat, and cold* may all be symptomatic, not so much of regression, but of disassociation from an external reality that is too confusing or painful to maintain contact with. In this manner, hallucinations and delusions involve mechanisms of denial first, and then projection of an internal state so as to reconstitute an imaginary world. Nonetheless, when analyzed, the imaginary world contains many elements from the denied and nonassimilated real world. This hallucinatory, delusional reconstitution protects the child from a more profound regression to autistic formlessness, chaos, or emptiness.

As we have seen earlier, *cognitive arrests* are symptomatic of the baby's inability to discriminate its effect upon inanimate and animate objects in the world and to gain a permanent image of them. Without such an image, purposeful and trial-and-error activity and speech are impossible because all require representations. In speech the representations are verbal symbols. To a significant extent, then, representational failure must be involved in *speech symptoms* in the second and third years of life. It must also be implicated in the antecedent symptom of *failure of facial expression to signify mood, intent, and meaning* at twelve months.

By contrast, *phobias* are symptoms in early life, as in adult life, that involve symbolic capacity. Using the primitive defense of displacement, the child shifts intense affects from one person, representation, experience, body function, or object to another in an effort to protect the former.

## Conclusion

Words can only approximate the developmental disturbances we have been describing. The baby who is the victim cannot testify on his own behalf since by age and illness his language is not equal to the task. Therefore we have had to construct from moving pictures, and reconstruct from therapy and histories, the baby's experience. This has led us to postulate a psychotogenic process that evolves from disturbances in the patterning of the parent-infant relationship across the bonding and attachment modalities of gazing, vocalizing, touching, holding, and affect.

Several mechanisms characterize the pathogenic effect of aberrant parent-infant interaction upon psychological development. These mechanisms are: (1) unpredictably discrepant and noncontingent parent or infant responses which violate turn-taking; (2) nonshared or nonconsummated affective interchange; (3) failures of parental empathy and misunderstandings of meanings; (4) parental frustration, overstimulation, and overcontrol of the infant; (5) dyssynchronous interactions in rhythm and force (intensity); and (6) paradoxical (contradictory, mutually exclusive, or double-binding) responses. In recognizing these mechanisms, we attempt to give meaning to phenomena we have observed. These forces are related, often describing closely connected aspects of similar events which cause a disengagement of parent and child from each other in terms of external behavior, as well as with respect to inner life. The levels of distinction are important, however, because each alerts us to different areas of infant developmental organization of internal state and external response which aberrant parent-infant interaction disrupts.

We theorize, supported by our case examples, that in a given family with severe psychopathology most of these mechanisms operate relatively continuously. They exert their destructive effect through the chronic pressure they impose on developmental processes. In addition, it is theoretically likely that the infant is particularly vulnerable to the traumatic effects of these mechanisms during periods of major transitions in development when a key neurological maturational step coincides with a significant advance in psychological growth. Data reviewed in Chapters 3 and 4 point to several of these junctures. There is the differentiation of sleep and wakefulness into day and night cycles in the first weeks of life which makes the baby more available to interaction with its caretakers; there is the transition from midbrain control of behavior to forebrain control of behavior (endogenous to exogenous control) which gives the infant greater flexibility and autonomy in response to stimuli than allowed by the prior, more reflex interactional entrainment with the parent; and there is the special smile for the mother at about three to four months which coincides with the infant's gaining the ability to distinguish configurations of features through targeting and processing images in the fovea of the retina.

Somewhat later there occur the major psychological events of stranger anxiety signifying advancing self-object discrimination and capacity for temporal anticipation; intersubjectivity, whereby the infant perceives that it not only has intentions but that two people can share an intention; and finally language, which indicates a capacity for symbol formation. These three later developmental steps probably also coincide with neurologic maturation, although the anatomical correlates have not been elucidated. All of the transitions bring the child into increasing interpersonal contact. At each of the developmental junctures, potentially pathogenic infant-parent interactions in the forms reviewed in this chapter, combined with chronicity of effect, may disorder the neurophysiologic substrate of behavior, the underlying basic psychological structures of the baby, and the patterning of the child's external behavior. Conversely, if the infant's neurologic maturation is inherently disordered, as Fish's data (1977) from the development of children of schizophrenic parents suggests may be the case in some babies, it may disrupt the very parental responses which facilitate psychological growth in the child.

Synthesizing empirical data and theory, we come to an overall hypothesis that for many prepsychotic children the early percepts of, and experiences with the parent are fraught with pain and confusion. This leads to defense behaviors to ward off the danger inherent in this contact. The defensive reactions close off sensory and motor modalities of interaction and the building up of self-animate object and self-inanimate object schema. Consequently, inadequate schema impair cognition and distort self-object differentiation. Primitive defenses persist to mediate between internal and external reality far longer than occurs in normal development, or are called into play during regressions when the child faces a stress. Ultimately, symptoms of psychosis appear, signaling the child's inability to manage developmental demands. The psychotogenic model elaborated here, then, is a construct of a linkage of disturbed parent-infant behavior and psychic structuralization on the many layers outlined in this chapter.

In the course of this task, the ill child's fate sounds grim. However, on an optimistic note, review of the children's follow-ups shows that approximately one-third of the cases in our series made a reasonably successful noninstitutional adaptation, and were at least partially self-sufficient and appropriately advanced in school. This is similar to the reports of others (Goldfarb et al., 1978). In addition, we are convinced, on the basis of our familiarity with children suffering autism and other early childhood psychoses who received treatment prior to the third birthday, that early intervention can prevent an entrenched syndrome.

Yet in spite of this encouragement, there is also the possibility that an extremely large number of infants undergo the severe developmental interferences discussed here without demonstrating symptoms in early childhood. Their adaptational strengths and defenses are adequate for a time. At a later point in youth or adulthood, however, a normative maturational pressure, such as heterosexual intimacy or the need to earn a living under difficult circumstances, overtaxes their fragile adaptation. A schizophrenic decompensation occurs, characterized by many of the symptoms of the childhood illness, but acted out on a much broader scale because of the motor and social sophistication of the older person. In this view, schizophrenic breaks after childhood are not new illnesses, but the outcome of imperfectly mastered developmental stages and impaired psychic structuralization in the first three years of life. Historically, dyadic parent-infant difficulties interfere with self-object differentiation and individuation, and the preschizophrenic person relies after infancy on a preponderance of primitive defense mechanisms. Under the impact of intense affects during a normative or unusual life crisis, the primitive defenses prove too weak, and the psychotic break with reality occurs.

If this theory is correct, it alerts us even more strongly to the importance of early recognition of parent-infant difficulties. Nonetheless, our science is imperfect, and it is not yet clear why and how a particular set of parent-infant circumstances lead in one family to adult schizophrenia, in another family to one of the childhood psychosis syndromes, and in still another to a child with a personality disorder. Nonetheless, it seems clear that a child who experiences the kinds of traumas we have delineated will suffer some distortion of psychological maturation.

*Chapter 11*

# The Treatment of Psychosis in the First Four Years of Life: An Integration of New Ideas and Past Experience

As thinking pertaining to the psychoses of early childhood and to normal development in the first years of life evolves, it is important to consider how new knowledge should affect the treatment of psychosis in very early life. In particular, we want to apply findings from the Early Natural History of Childhood Psychosis Project to formulating a set of criteria for the assessment and treatment of children who fail to gain a sense of reality or who lose touch with reality in the first four years of life. Diagnostically they suffer from autism, symbiotic psychosis of childhood and mixed forms of early childhood psychosis.

New understanding of normal development as well as pathological growth has been insufficiently updated into an integrated theory of treatment in the past decade. This lag in advancing therapeutics critically hampers progress in healing during the first four years of life when illness can be most effectively treated, or even aborted in some children. Some of the pertinent issues are addressed in the recent review article by Shafii (1979) on the treatment of children suffering psychosis. Yet he omits consideration of some key developmental issues, such as Mahler's elucidation of the normal stages of separation and individuation. In addition, the author does not analyze contradictions inherent in some of the therapeutic strategies he discusses, such as the potential punitive effect on the child of negative reinforcement in behavior modification, which is counter to the emphasis on building a bond through trust between therapist and patient, which is a cornerstone of psychodynamic therapeutic theory. Before Shafii's review, we must go back to Szurek and Berlin's *Clinical Studies in Childhood Psychosis* (1973). This comprehensive volume addresses issues that Shafii omits, but it did not have available to it the work of the past ten to fifteen years. In this chapter we propose an approach to the treatment of psychotic conditions in the first four years of life that incorporates recent advances in development and therapeutics. Our approach is based on the elaboration of nine basic criteria for planning treatment of early childhood psychosis and autism. These nine elements, phrased as questions, guide both the assessment of children and the conduct of treatment.

## Nine Guidelines to the Treatment of Autism and Psychosis in Early Childhood

1. Has a specific organic demonstrable condition, such as a brain lesion, metabolic, neurophysiological, or infectious process, been ruled out?
2. What is the nature of the child's relationships with people (i.e., the child's attachments)?
3. What is the nature of the parent-child interaction?
4. Are the parents able to participate in the child's treatment?
5. In what stage of separation and individuation is the child?
6. What are the recurring conscious and unconscious fantasies of the child in relation to people (the major objects in his life) and things? Is the child's fantasy and instinctual life largely oral, anal, sadistic, incorporative, expulsive, inchoate, or fragmented? Are fantasies and urges profoundly repressed, directed outward, or somaticized and self-directed?
7. At what stage of sensorimotor cognitive development, in Piaget's scheme, is the child? And if beyond this level, what kinds of preoperational tasks can he or she perform?
8. What indications are there for behavior modification?
9. What indications are there for pharmacotherapy?

A case example will illustrate how our approach to treatment is built around these nine questions. Following the narration of the child's clinical history is a discussion of the nine points as they apply to this child and how they can be generalized to other patients.

## Case Example

### HISTORY

Helen was three-and-a-half years old when she was referred for diagnosis and treatment by her daycare center because she neither spoke nor socialized with other children. At the initial screening it was evident that Helen's development was severely disturbed and that her unmarried mother was so overwhelmed by her daughter's problems that she was not able to come to the clinic consistently. Therefore, Helen entered a children's inpatient psychiatric unit for evaluation and the beginning of treatment. Neurologic studies and medical tests did not reveal any biological abnormalities. While hospitalized, she participated in a therapeutic milieu that included activities with other children, companionship with a consistent nurse, thrice weekly play therapy with a child psychiatrist, and conjoint sessions with her mother and the psychiatrist. The conjoint sessions occurred at infrequent intervals, averaging about one a month, because the mother cancelled more frequent sessions.

Attempts to engage the mother in therapy for herself were also unsuccessful. The unit social worker did learn from the mother, however, that Helen was conceived out of wedlock with a man the mother disliked. The mother considered having an abortion but decided to maintain the pregnancy. Nonetheless, when Helen was born the mother experienced a feeling of revulsion. She felt the child looked like an animal at first, and later felt that the baby resembled the disliked father. The mother recalled her severe depression during the child's first year, and she frequently enlisted others to care for the child from birth to the present although she remained the principal caretaker. The mother's work record was not good, and she volunteered that she drank too much. She could not recall ever having loved the child, and she felt that Helen, on her part, had never responded affectionately to her.

### DESCRIPTION OF THE CHILD AND RELATIONSHIP TO THE MOTHER

Helen herself was diagnosed as autistic but intermittently available for interaction. The child had been toilet-trained for about a year, and fed herself awkwardly with utensils. She used no words and was echolalic. She frequently expressed herself with loud whines when excited, grunts whenever she wanted something, and screams when angry—largely the repertoire of a nine-to-sixteen-month-old child. Her expression was often grimacing, and she avoided eye contact. She did not play with children and shrank back when people approached her. Often screaming at these moments, she ran to her room and engaged in stereotypies—rocking, head banging, waving her hands in front of her face, and running water from a sink or toilet over her hands. Nonetheless, in spite of her withdrawal and isolation people still existed for Helen as indexed by her curiosity about them and attraction to them. For example, when left alone Helen stood at the periphery of the children watching intently. She could also be seen gazing intently at the back of a staff person, sometimes smiling shyly but winsomely, and this made her a staff favorite.

In early observations of Helen and her mother, the child remained relatively frozen in the mother's presence with an unhappy tense expression. She obeyed compliantly. Neither mother nor child showed any pleasure in the other, and both were wooden. The only spontaneous expressions were the mother's harsh commands and exasperated criticisms, "do that . . . don't . . . why can't you . . . hurry up!"

### THE COURSE OF THERAPY

Helen remained hospitalized for nine months, during which time the ward staff and children became her surrogate family. After several initial weeks she no longer panicked when staff approached. She began to smile coquettishly, averting her gaze only when they came close, while offering her hand to be held, especially to her psychiatrist and her regular nurse. When walking, she followed a pace back and to the side of people. All of the pronounced stereotypies and behavioral symptoms diminished, emerging intensely only when Helen was tired, frustrated, or felt coerced.

Helen's individual treatment three times weekly for an hour provided the clearest description of her illness. At first she was aloof and avoidant of her doctor. Yet her self-imposed isolation was painful, for she also wanted to form an attachment as indicated by her shy glances and adherence to a territorial or geographic periphery that allowed some, but not complete, separation from the therapist. The doctor was availably affectionate and parental, staying as close to Helen as she would allow during the initial months of treatment.

The doctor encouraged Helen to go on walks and spend time in the playroom with her, and she followed her to her room when Helen retreated. Their relationship was largely one of parallel behaviors: Helen engaged in repetitive stereotyped activities which the therapist imitated, all the while providing Helen with the words for the names of objects and verbalizing what was going on between the two of them. The doctor added how she, as therapist, felt, and wondered how Helen felt. Helen never responded with words. The therapist tried to introduce variations into activities or to elaborate the repetitive play into a story that the child might pursue alone or with the doctor—again to no avail early in treatment. Occasionally the therapist had to retreat physically or hold Helen firmly if she became too excited or endangered property, by flooding the room, for example, or threatened herself with head banging.

After about six months there was a distinct change in the child. She began greeting her doctor and nurse with genuine and increasing enthusiasm by running into their arms to be picked up, and smiling and squealing with pleasure. She maintained visual contact for seconds at a time. Her vocalizations began to have the cadence and intonation of speech, and she began to point at objects and people in connection with special sounds she made to signify her recognition of them as well as to indicate wishes. We now understood that Helen had developed a psychological attachment to the most important people in her current life, which formerly had either not existed or had been warded off by the mother and child to the point of nonexistence. Thus when her therapist or nurse were away on vacation, Helen's mood changed and she became resistant. She was irritable, engaged in more repetitive behaviors, and was less in contact with people. When her surrogate family returned, she quickly reentered her new affectionate relationship with them. We inferred from this that the child had established a benign mental representation of her nurse and doctor as human beings separate from herself. Their absences were painful to Helen, but they did not destroy the child's capacity to reenter her relationship with them as caring people on their return.

At the same time Helen began to greet her mother with spontaneous smiles and looks. The mother, in spite of encouragement to participate as frequently as possible, came to the hospital only approximately once in two weeks during this phase of treatment. Equally perniciously, she did not seem to be able to perceive her child's greetings and attempts at contact. Even with guidance, coaching, and attempts at personal exploration, the mother habitually turned to the doctor to talk *about* Helen just as Helen approached her, criticizing what she felt was her daughter's coldness towards her and lack of improvement. In turn, at these moments of rebuff, Helen became confused. Her expressions then reverted toward her frozen compliance to her mother, and she transiently became wooden and compliant toward the hospital staff.

Because of the mother's unresponsiveness to treatment (and with the mother's concurrence), plans were made to discharge Helen to nurturing foster parents who would continue to bring the child to her psychiatrist for thrice weekly outpatient sessions. This took place after nine months of treatment when it seemed that attachment to and mental representation of the doctor were solid. At the time of admission to the hospital, Helen had given no indication that she could distinguish between inner feelings and external events; but during her months in the therapeutic milieu she had progressed to a brief symbiotic attachment to her therapist, and thence to the beginning of psychological separation and individuation, as Mahler has outlined. Behaviors such as the child's pleasurable clinging to the therapist and her inability to signify wishes by gesture or word, while depending upon her therapist to understand and meet her needs, were consistent with the phase of Helen's symbiotic tie to the therapist in which there was little differentiation between self and other. By contrast, Helen signified her emergence from this phase to separation and individuation through her sense of loss when her principal staff members were away, and her pleasurable recognition of them on their return which bespoke her mental representation of them as distinct from her self-representation. Also indicative of separation and individuation was her development of a gestural and vocal vocabulary for objects as clearly distinct from herself. She began to experiment with different functions of objects and accept at times suggestions from her doctor to play with particular toys. Thus by four years and three months of age, Helen had reached the emotional level of approximately twelve months. In addition, her strong curiosity about people and children led us to feel confident that at this point there was a powerful, healthy developmental drive toward mastery and human relationships. This would lead Helen towards relative normalcy as long as she had a primary relationship with her therapist to facilitate the drive, to protect Helen from external interferences by insuring that her home was a nurturing one, and to provide the context for recognizing the emergence of any specific disturbing fantasies that might require corrective interpretation in play sessions.

In terms of her cognitive capacity, at three-and-a-half years of age during her first months in the hospital, Helen functioned largely at the level of what Piaget had described as primary and secondary circular reactions (sensorimotor stages 2 and 3, normally seen between two and ten months). That is, her behaviors were repetitive motor actions with her hands, mouth, or whole body acting upon themselves (primary circular reactions) and not upon other people or things, or repetitive manipulations of objects, such as the toilet handle or a toy, to make an interesting spectacle last (secondary circular reactions). At the same time, however, Helen had also learned and maintained the skill of eating with utensils. This is a sensorimotor stage 5 level of cognitive function demonstrating Helen's connection of the means by which one eats (the spoon) with the ends (ingestion). Likewise the child's use of the toilet signifies her mental capacity to connect a physical sensation with the use of an object. Gradually we observed Helen broaden her repertoire and range of interests so that her thought was clearly more complex and less rigid as the primary and secondary reactions diminished. Door and drawer mechanisms interested her, and manipulation of pencils and crayons to make lines and colors, though without recognizable shapes, appeared. She learned to enjoy recognizing the connection between parts of toys and their functions. All of this indicated, as months passed, a primitive but mentally informed curiosity that normal children typically show in the second half of the first year of life and in the second year. In Helen, it was appearing in the fourth year of life.

A major cognitive breakthrough occurred in the seventh to ninth month of hospitalization, just prior to discharge. It was complimentary to and simultaneous with Helen's emotional advances of psychological attachment, mental representation of her therapist, and beginning separation of her own self-representation from that of her therapist. Helen began to demonstrate acute perception of where objects were moved to when they were displaced from her view in play or rearranged in her room, indicating nascent object permanence (sensorimotor stages 4 and 5, normally seen between ten and eighteen months). Of equal import in the emotional realm, was the appearance of transient panic states during this time. As Helen both accepted closeness to her doctor and took her doctor's presence more for granted, she played for longer periods of time with objects in an exploratory rather than compulsively stereotypic way while her therapist kept her company. Helen would also cruise alone from the playroom into the hallways and then return. Suddenly she might panic and start screaming as if frightened, wave her hands in front of her face, and lean against her doctor or sit in her doctor's lap until calmed—either spontaneously or with the doctor's forceful urging. We understood this as a rapprochement subphase, in Mahler's scheme, normally appearing between fourteen and twenty-two months, but in Helen at close to four-and-a-half years, which was almost nine months after treatment began.

The subphase signifies the threat the child feels to its mental image of the mother and its own self-image. Both of these images are not yet consolidated, but they are sufficiently robust to give the child courage to play independently until separation from the parent figure threatens the self and object representation. The frightened toddler then quickly returns to make concrete tactile contact with the mother. Yet it also fears the regressive pull toward merger with the mother, so that, caught between the wish for autonomy and the fear of it, the child darts away and back for a period of time. We predicted that, if this were in fact a rapprochement subphase, it would pass in a few weeks, and we would next see Helen showing the first signs of symbol formation, as normally occurs toward the end of the second year of life.

Helen did gratify us by soon bringing dolls into her play for the first time. She treated them as representations of herself and how she wished to be treated. She also treated them like other little people, cuddling and grooming them in a way that showed that Helen had achieved the capacity to use one thing (a doll) to stand for another (a human being). To make use of representations is inherent in the simple function of words that stand for actions, things, and feelings. Nonetheless, Helen did not yet have a spoken language. At the same time, Helen began to enjoy being groomed by her nurse and doctor, she took pleasure in picking out clothes, and she tried to comb her own hair and point out her own and her doctor's body parts in games—all indicating a solidification of her body image as having a form and identity of its own, a phenomenon normally occurring in the second to third years, occurring in this little girl in the fifth year.

During these advances, Helen left the hospital for her foster home. The transition was surprisingly smooth. Now that symbolization and representational thought had been achieved, Helen for the first time told stories in her play with dolls during her outpatient therapy sessions, stories which gave expression to her fantasy life. They were simple enactments of people coming and going without strong affective qualities, suggesting that they were Helen's attempts to master her own losses by turning passive experiences into active experiences. These were the loss of her mother when the mother was emotionally unavailable to Helen; the real loss of the mother when the child moved into the hospital; and the departure from her hospital family. Further, her newly developed self-identity and perception of her therapist as a stable object representation (both distilled from an earlier self-object matrix) must have felt to Helen as fragile and vulnerable to aggression and erasure. We suspected that, in addition to loss, this lingering fragility was being mastered by Helen in her doll play of people coming and going. At this point, the doctor could verbally interpret to the child her fears of loss and helplessness, interpretations to which Helen listened intently.

## Discussion

The technical aspects of treatment in Helen's case were narrated in the clinical presentation. However, examining the nine guidelines for planning and conducting treatment in early childhood psychosis and autism, as they apply to Helen, makes explicit our thinking for all the major therapeutic decisions in the case. A profile of the child emerges which illustrates how similar profiles can be constructed for other severely disturbed children in a manner analogous to Anna Freud's Diagnostic Profile (1962) for more general developmental issues.

1. *Has a specific demonstrable condition, such as a brain lesion, metabolic, neurophysiological, or infectious process, been ruled out?* For Helen the answer was affirmative. Whenever a child shows bizarre behavior, it is essential to rule out a central-nervous-system-affecting intoxication, metabolic condition, space-occupying tumor, infection, or injury. Treatment of such demonstrable lesions can often be rapid and life-saving. This is in contrast to the field's current active investigation into possible metabolic, genetic, traumatic, and even infectious etiologies of the early childhood psychoses (Ritvo et al., 1976). In these areas, research has not yet been able to isolate a specific pathognomonic factor or structural abnormality which is proven to have been premorbid rather than a consequence of the illness. In the absence of such evidence, we choose to view the use of metabolic substances (e.g., L-dopamine) or anatomic manipulation (e.g., vestibular stimulation) as investigational and nonspecific. Therefore we avoid the use of these approaches in the clinical nonresearch endeavor. Nonetheless, such treatment may on occasion effect symptoms in a way that is

similar to the effect that phenothiazines and other major tranquilizers sometimes have on behavior. In this regard, we return to the question of symptom control with a discussion of points 8 and 9 below.

2. *What is the nature of the child's relationship with people (i.e., its attachments)?* Helen was extremely isolated from everyone including her mother when treatment began. She desparately avoided eye contact and physical closeness, and did not speak. People's absences brought no response from her. From the referring day-care agency, we knew this had been the case for at least the past year, and the mother felt it had characterized Helen's behavior from infancy. Behaviorally, we could speak of Helen as unattached. However, intrapsychically, even as treatment was beginning, she had a psychological attachment to people, albeit a bond whose quality was conflicted and highly ambivalent. This was evident in her curious glances at people when she felt they were not looking at her and in the distance she kept—not too far nor too close—from hospital staff and her mother. Whether she was trying to escape a pain inherent in too much proximity, or trying to overcome isolation by coming closer, we could not tell. But we could infer that Helen's mental images of her mother and other people were distorted by affects of confusion, fear, rage, and longing associated with these people. Distance from social contact seemed to attenuate these emotions. The source of Helen's distortions of reality is uncertain. But whatever the cause, in order to understand her object relationships fully we also had to consider the next question.

3. *What is the nature of the parent-child interaction?* We observed the mother's reluctance to approach Helen, her critical, cool expression with the child, her verbal dislike of the child, and her turning away from Helen's gaze and smile to address the doctor instead. For a disturbed child, such maternal behaviors must reinforce the child's sense of isolation and its helplessness in drawing close. Further, the mother's aversive response must create in the child confusion, because the expected contingent response to the child's developing communication of a wish for affiliation through smiling is not forthcoming from the parent. The isolation, helplessness, and confusion are affective states which potentially breed the aforementioned rage which we inferred must be part of Helen's internal object representations. They are also affective states that contribute to her ambivalence and distortions of reality.

This assessment of Helen's object relations and of her interactions with her mother establishes that the first priorities of treatment are to reduce the child's isolation and to establish a strong and benignly experienced attachment between the patient and another human being. Our first choice is to use the parents to accomplish this attachment through counselling them so that they become our therapeutic allies, if not the principal therapists themselves. Treating through the parents may have three advantages: it builds on the parents' own bond to the child; the parents are not strangers to the patient; and the parents may be able to spend many more hours a week working with the child than professional therapists can.

Vivid accounts of parents establishing or reestablishing an enduring affectionate attachment with their autistic children, which made possible subsequent healthy growth, are given by Clancy and McBride (1969) and Kaufman (1976). Clancy and McBride described therapy in Australia in which parents and the ill child are hospitalized together for several weeks so that the professional staff can intensively support and instruct the family in vigilant self-observation against behaviors which reinforce a child's withdrawal, as well as in ways to make contact with the child. The Kaufmans, because of frustration with the seeming futility of the professional treatment they encountered, instinctively and empathically developed a treatment for their young autistic son which is similar in orientation to what we have described in our case report of Helen and to what Clancy and McBride propose. With dedication and resourcefulness far beyond the physical, economic, and emotional capacity that most families can muster on their own, parents and siblings spent hours in daily shifts playing in parallel with the Kaufman child. They intruded physically into his gaze and verbally into his isolation, holding him close and trying to entrain each glimmer of a response or initiatory behavior he made into a human reciprocal relationship. Finally their efforts paid off with responses similar to Helen's, so that the child first formed an interpersonal tie, then proceeded to separate emotionally and individuate.

However, before deciding to embark on such a course of therapy that instrumentally involves the parents, we need to consider whether they are capable of this role. Guideline 4 addresses this question.

4. *Are the parents able to participate in the child's treatment?* In the face of her daughter's illness and rejecting behavior (even though Helen gradually became responsive), Helen's mother was not herself responsive to counselling that sought to help her initiate a friendly approach to her child. For this reason, it was necessary to use hospital treatment initially, and later to enlist foster parents who could be therapeutic allies of the child's psychiatrist. Had the mother been able

to overcome her own hurt and angry withdrawal from her daughter, the patient might have been able to return home after treatment had progressed, and then continue in clinic or day treatment. And, if the mother had been able to participate in treatment rapidly and productively, it might have been possible to avoid hospitalizing Helen and to treat the child on an intensive outpatient basis. But this was not the case, and we felt that our therapeutic efforts with Helen were being undone during the time she spent with her mother. When the parents are unable to act therapeutically for the child, the therapist functions as a surrogate parent, drawing the child out of its isolation and into a human attachment. In slow steps, the child cautiously tests itself as a separate entity while feeling the support of its caretaker.

5. *At what stage of separation and individuation is the child?* At admission we documented Helen's initial autistic (presymbiotic) stage, and then followed her up the developmental ladder of separation and individuation. Chronicling this progress is the most useful indication of the efficacy of the child's treatment. It verified that Helen was advancing in identity formation and in relatedness to the people in her life. By contrast, following only the wax and wane of symptoms such as stereotypies or grimacing tells the therapist little about where the child stands in relation to normal development since a child may be without signs of bizarreness but still be symbiotically tied (in the sense of intrapsychic development) to the mother.

When we first noted progress in Helen's psychological development, we were very optimistic that there existed a potential for growth. We felt that the drive for development now functioning would continue to carry Helen emotionally unless either external traumas or internal biological factors interfered. For example, it is hypothesized but not proven that a genetic factor may result in an enzymatic abnormality that affects central nervous system neurotransmitters and, consequently, behavior. Such an enzyme defect may be present at birth or arise later in the child's life. Therefore, as therapists we conceptualized that an important part of our role was to be alert to potential new interferences in the child's development. Biology did not interfere—it only aided growth in a normal fashion in Helen's case. And with respect to protection against environmental trauma, as we said, we arranged for the child to leave the hospital in the care of responsive foster parents who facilitated the girl's normalization.

6. *What are the recurring conscious and unconscious fantasies of the child in relation to people and things?* Fantasies are fed by and fuel the child's

instinctual life and defensive functioning, so we also ask what characterizes the child's instinctual life? Further, what are the child's defenses? These arise from and organize interpersonal experience; they also provide intrapsychic structure. Is the child's mental life largely oral, anal, sadistic, incorporative, expulsive, fragmented, or profoundly repressed? For example, with respect to primitive repression, has the child, in Mahler's term (1968), "de-animated" the self and object world, leaving both lifeless? Or has the patient possibly somaticized and self-directed aggression, as occurs in self-starvation or self-mutilation?

The treatment of psychotic children requires answering these questions. As P. Kernberg has recently written (1980), therapy

> implies a task of deciphering components of self and object, as they are fragmented, bizarre, projected, or introjected in the most unexpected combinations; and of exploring primitive fantasies to render them accessible to interpersonal sharing and secondary process (pp. 615–616).

For example, Kernberg describes a five-year-old schizophrenic boy who rubbed paint, glue, and water on his therapist's and mother's skin. The child's fantasy was that this action would erase the traumatic and primitive ego fragmenting, and the unbearable threatening separateness between himself and those who were "not him." Further, in our experience a five-year-old suffering symbiotic psychosis of childhood refused to eat away from home (Case 4 in the Childhood Psychosis Project). He had the delusion that any food prepared by someone other than his mother was poison. This delusion was a consequence of the intense closeness between the mother and patient, as well as the mother's projections onto the child of her own fears of loss and her guilt over separation from the baby. Therapeutically, understanding the fantasies produced by children such as these and then giving words to the previously silent, unconscious, or simply acted out ideas is the first step in helping patients to understand their own distortions of reality and master them.

On the other hand, in our case example Helen did not produce evidence of specific and powerfully disorganizing pathological fantasies akin to those just described. Rather, at the beginning of hospitalization Helen seemed to be in a state of detachment—perhaps deanimation—where there was no stable representation or discrete sensory experience of inner and outer life nor of herself as distinct from others. Therapeutically, we first had to reconnect for her these pieces of experience; or, if they had never existed in an integrated fashion—a real possibility—we had to allow the pieces to coalesce into the formation of, first, a symbiotic human tie and, then, a separate identity. When this latter degree of psychological structuralization is present—generally in the second and third years of life, but in Helen appearing at about four-and-a-half years—the child has an image of the self and objects as distinct from the self, with rapidly increasing stability of representation. Contemporaneously, the capacity for symbol formation occurs, the sine qua non of speech. At this stage there is sufficient psychological structuralization for fantasy life, conscious and unconscious dichotomies, and defense mechanisms. All are accessible through play, stories, or verbally to both patient and therapist. Treatment with Helen had just reached this point as our case narration drew to a close, with the appearance of doll-play stories that represented many layers of emotional experience. Prior to this, mental life had been ineffable and unformed, characterized by primitive mental processes and defenses such as fragmentation, introjection, and projection, and, in children with beginning illness, primitive defense behaviors such as "turning away."

7. *At what specific stage of Piagetian cognitive development is the child? What sensorimotor level has been reached, and can the child perform any preoperational tasks?* Cognitive capacity and emotional growth are much more closely intertwined than had been previously thought when Freud's and Piaget's systems were viewed as belonging to two distinct realms of life. Greenspan (1979) charts how affective disturbances can impinge upon a child's ability to construct a picture of the world through sensory and motor experience and upon a child's ability to classify, conserve, and think about propositions. Reasoning helps one order the world of human relations. With a child less than four years of age who is suffering an early childhood psychosis, we are specifically concerned with sensorimotor cognition. Advanced sensorimotor achievements are the child's ability to know that an object has an existence even when it is not present (object permanence) and that one thing can be used to represent an absent object (symbolization). Generally occurring at the end of the second year and in the third year of life, these phenomena are contemporaneous with the child's gaining of libidinal object constancy, as Mahler has described the last step in the separation-individuation sequence. By this time the child holds in mind an image of the mother that is relatively firm, even in her physical absence, relatively accurately endowed with the range of her qualities as experienced by the child, and distinct from

the child's self-representation. However, if an infant has had separations from the mother, personal injuries or illnesses that distort the experience of the body, or traumatic interactional experiences with the mother (e.g., of the kind described in Helen's case which affect attachment and differentiation), libidinal object constancy is disturbed. There are also increasing indications that these events then exert a pathogenic or "spillover" effect on nonhuman object permanence (Greenspan, 1979). For example, at the beginning of treatment at three-and-a-half years, Helen showed primarily stage 2 and 3 behaviors which suggested that her cognitive world was largely body-centered and was without objects as we know them. Gradually people and things took shape and had recognizable properties that she learned to integrate into her cognitive functioning and to manipulate physically and mentally. She also learned how to identify the way people and things produced sensations in her, how to interact with them, how to anticipate events and responses, and how to discern predictable and nonpredictable patterns in their behavior.

Therapy must not make cognitive demands on the psychotic patient which are more than a step beyond the grasp of the child. For example, it would have been fruitless to expect Helen to know the name of her doctor, to know that the doctor would not hurt her, and to anticipate the hour of the doctor's arrival, or to miss the doctor during vacations *before* she began to have an early image of the doctor as a distinct entity. Such an image corresponds to the shift from symbiosis to beginning separation-individuation in the second six months of life in the normal child. In Helen it also occurred after about six months of treatment, but at the age of four years.

Strategically in our treatment of young psychotic children it seems helpful to build in mild cognitive complexities and emotional frustrations that are nontraumatic and nondisorganizing, but which lead the child to higher stages of reasoning and increase the child's ability to postpone gratification and manage anger without withdrawal. This is an effective paradigm also for adjunctive educational therapists to follow. Efforts which bolster cognitive processes—*as distinct from* rote teaching of information and vocabulary building that does not take into account how the child can use information—facilitate how the child makes sense of the people in its life. Demands for comprehension that are beyond the child's capacity may also trigger panic attacks or confused regression because of the patient's developmental lag in structuralizing mechanisms, such as adequate defenses, for the modulation of affects.

8. *What indications are there for behavior modification?* We are very

cautious about employing behavior modification in autism and other early childhood psychoses, and reserve it for the specific control of acute symptoms which are life-threatening and unresponsive to the psychodynamic and psychoanalytically derived efforts so far described.

The only physically dangerous symptom Helen exhibited was head banging, and this never reached unremitting severity. Further, within weeks of hospitalization the symptom became less frequent and intense, reserved by Helen for moments of great tension. Likewise, the child's general isolation and unsocialized behaviors responded slowly but steadily to the therapeutic approach already described.

Our caution with behavior modification grows from the fact that some behavioral techniques establish a patient-therapist interaction which recreates or parallels the very failures of emotional reciprocity that existed between the autistic child and her parents. Failure of emotional reciprocity was clearly the case with Helen. For example, behavior modification attempts to "extinguish" nonsocial or dangerous target behaviors through aversive stimuli, which may be in the form of physical pain or punishment, or in the form of the therapist's withdrawing reinforcers of undesirable actions from the child. This may be done by the therapist's ignoring unwanted behavior, and through withdrawing smiles, praise, affection, and body contact from the patient when the child is showing unwanted symptoms. When the patient behaves in an appropriate fashion, the therapist will attempt to selectively reward the child with reinforcers which are pleasing, such as smiles, approbation, and food. However, Helen had received no smiles at all for an indeterminate period because the mother found all of the child's actions undesirable. If the therapy recreated an ambience of selective affection and coldness, it would oppose our goal of establishing an attachment between the child and people which was not heavily laced with the ambivalence that aversive stimuli and negative reinforcers produce. Our understanding of the intrapsychic life of the psychotic child, as already described, suggests that it is replete with ambivalence because of the confusion, inconsistency, and fragmented affects of rage and pleasure that the human and object worlds have for the patient. Therefore, therapists must be extremely careful about adding further sources of ambivalence to the child's life.

In addition, we are concerned that many of the socializing behaviors which behavior modification "shapes" for the disturbed child are not truly integrated into the child's development of self- and object constancy. For example, a stereotypie can be extinguished, and a social greeting created in an autistic child. But what is the emotional significance of this if the child has not yet achieved a representation of itself that is distinct and a representation of another person that is nonfragmented? Behavior modification training for such a patient may be akin to toilet training a child prematurely at one year. At this age a child has no conception of body parts and a very shaky mental representation of body sensations. The outcome of the regimented training in either situation, prior to the child's cognitive and affective readiness, may be children who are automatons with little capacity to think and feel.

9. *What indications are there for pharmacotherapy?* Administering pharmacological agents in the early childhood psychoses need not have the same potentially dangerous effect on interpersonal interactions as behavior modification. Nonetheless, we are also cautious with psychotropic medicines because of several considerations. Symptoms such as avoidant behaviors may serve an important defensive function for the child. Therefore we avoid premature attempts to cut off such behavior until the child has been psychologically prepared to lose the defenses certain symptoms provide, and until traumatic caretaking has been mitigated so that the child is less at risk emotionally and therefore less in need of its accustomed ways of dealing with interpersonal experiences. Likewise, we are also concerned that the central nervous system effects of powerful pharmacologic agents may potentially interfere with certain intrapsychic developmental accomplishments such as the child's achieving self-object discrimination and the consolidation of schema and representations. With these considerations in mind, we reserve medications for instances of physically dangerous symptoms, such as assaultive or self-destructive behavior, and manifestations of psychosis, such as intractible withdrawal, which do not respond to psychodynamic-psychoanalytically informed treatment.

Operating within this guideline, Helen did not receive medication. If she had not responded as she did, however, we would have considered a trial of medication such as chlorpromazine (Thorazine), trifluperazine (Stelazine), or butyrophenone (Haldol). It is unclear whether these drugs are specific for a possible pathologic lesion underlying psychosis and what their mechanism of action is. Nonetheless, the medications have empirically been shown to be useful in some children for the symptomatic control of agitation, hallucinations, delusions, and destructive behavior.

**TABLE 11-1** *Steps in the Treatment of Psychotic Conditions in Children Under 4 Years of Age*

1. Rule out specific organic demonstrable conditions such as infectious processes, tumors, and epilepsy.
2. Determine whether (and how) the child is psychologically attached to its parents and other people.
3. Describe the parent-child interaction.
4. Ascertain if the parents are able to respond to therapeutic help and modify pathologic responses to the child so as to be able to participate in the child's treatment.
5. Establish an emotional bond between child and therapist; and between child and parents (or surrogate parents if the parents are not able to be therapeutic allies).
6. Follow the child's progress in treatment through identifying it's progress through the stages of psychological separation and individuation (from autism to symbiosis to beginning separation to the practicing subphase to the rapprochement subphase to self and object differentiation and libidinal object constancy).
7. When the child is able to express fantasies through play or verbally, identify the child's recurring conscious and unconscious fantasies in relation to people, things, and the therapist. Is the child's fantasy and instinctual life largely oral, anal, sadistic, incorporative, expulsive, inchoate, or fragmented? Are the fantasies and urges profoundly repressed, directed outward, or somaticized and self-directed?
8. Identify and follow the child's mastery of the sensorimotor stages of cognitive development; correlate the attainment of libidinal object constancy with object permanence, and with the child's capacity for symbolization (to make one thing stand for another) through language or play. Cognitive expectations in therapy should not be more than one step ahead of the child's cognitive attainments.
9. Reserve behavior modification for intractible physically dangerous symptoms.
10. Reserve medications for physically dangerous symptoms, anxiety, and hallucinations and delusions which appear intractible with verbal therapy.

# Conclusion •

The guidelines for framing treatment in the early childhood psychoses are independent of the etiology of the illness. Rather, for effective treatment the emphasis is on the recognition of illness very early and the therapist's use of an understanding of the patient's progress through psychological separation and individuation to guide therapeutic goals through each stage. As A. Freud (1962) has written,

> . . . neither symptomatology nor life tasks can be taken as reliable guides to the assessment of mental health or illness in childhood. . . . It is the diagnostician's task to ascertain where a given child stands on the developmental scale, whether his position is age adequate, retarded or precocious, and in what extent the observable internal and external circumstances and existent symptoms are interfering with . . . future growth (p. 150).

In this manner, understanding the developmental appropriateness of the child's cognitive maturation, object relations, fantasy life, and parent-child interactions also guide therapy. The framework presented in this chapter also assists the therapist in evaluating the place of behavior modification, medications, other somatic therapies, and in-home or out-of-home treatment in any therapeutic program.

Therapy does not always progress as propitiously as it did for Helen, even when conducted within the framework presented in this chapter, and even when treatment begins early in life. It has been our experience that Helen, coming to treatment at three-and-a-half years of age, was at the upper limit of the age when an autistic syndrome can be aborted or resolved. Even prior to age 4, an additional factor that is significant in the prognosis is the length of time the child has suffered severe symptoms. After four years with autistic children, therapeutic gains have been limited to specific areas of functioning and interpersonal relating. The prognosis for the syndromes of mixed forms of early childhood psychosis and symbiotic psychosis of childhood continues to be favorable even after four years with the intensive mixed cognitive and psychoanalytic developmentally oriented strategies outlined here.

However after infancy and toddler-hood the treatment of autism *per se* is still highly experimental. An approach emphasizing psychodynamics is clearly not sufficient to produce a predictably favorable outcome. For older children we would begin to focus increasing attention on their language and cognitive deficits and abilities in order to define their particular difficulties with concept and symbol formation, which is typically ridden with severe over-generalizations (parts of an idea or thing stand for wholes) and under-generalizations (wholes stand for only parts of an idea or thing). Whatever the contribution of earlier interpersonal phenomena to the syndrome, by a certain age (which seems to be variable but generally between two and four), the autistic child's ability to communicate with spoken or gestural language has become reified into a specific developmental failure. It has broken off from human object relations, and the ego and defense structuralization lines of development. Thus human contact may improve with psychodynamically oriented treatment of older children while language does not; and conversely language may at times outstrip the child's affective capacities. For these older children a behaviorally and linguistically oriented approach as described by Fay and Schuler (1980) may prove especially useful. The therapist identifies the child's conceptual difficulties, and then painstakingly attempts to give the child symbols in the form of sign language or spoken words to express ideas that the patient heretofore had no way to order and concretize in a form that made communication possible.

Finally, psychotropic medications also frequently have a more salutary effect and play a greater role in controlling symptoms and facilitating verbal treatment in children over four years of age.

# Appendix:
# The Massie-Campbell Scale of Mother-Infant Attachment Indicators During Stress

The Attachment During Stress Scale (ADS Scale) is a one-page guide to a standardized observation of components of mother-infant interaction for the pediatric clinician or mental health worker. The scale is composed of succinct descriptions of key parameters of mother-infant bonding—gazing, affective sharing, vocalizing, touching, infant clinging and maternal holding, and physical proximity—which are graded for the intensity of the attraction or avoidance between mother and baby and which are indicative of the adequacy or inadequacy of the mother's and baby's responsiveness. The principal purpose of this documentation is to assist the practitioner in the early identification of and therapeutic intervention with those families showing evidence of aberrant mother-infant interaction, in order to prevent the crystallization of pathological patterns of behavior and possible subsequent psychiatric illness in the child. The Scale can be used in any setting where mother and baby are together; however, a mild stress such as a well-baby physical examination or a mother-child reunion after separation heightens the interactions of mother and child, which makes the behaviors more evident for the observer.

Therefore the pediatric office or child-care center is an ideal place to apply the scale, which is designed for use with babies from birth until eighteen months of age.

## Background

### The Application of Recent Infancy Research

Three streams of clinical and research experience of the past several years have converged in the evolution of the Scale. The first has been the great increment over the past twenty years in knowledge of infant behavior and capacities. It was previously believed that the first months of a child's life consisted largely of physical growth and very little if any mental awareness. The parents were thought to structure reality for the baby, to control his environment, and to shape his behavior (Watson, 1926; Skinner, 1953). Consistent with this view was the sentiment that if the baby turned into a less than perfect child it was the parents' fault. Now it is recognized that the healthy neonate can focus his eyes and follow a human face, which he prefers over other objects (Fantz, 1965; Fantz & Miranda, 1975; Spitz, 1965). Although newborns habituate to excessive noise, they also hear and attend to voices (Klaus & Kennell, 1976; Brazelton, 1973), move their arms and legs synchronously with the rhythm of a speaker's voice (Condon & Sander, 1974), and smile and frown in response to pleasant or distressing events (Brazelton, 1973). The baby also often responds with quieting to gentle touch as well as with more oxygen uptake into the bloodstream when the mother touches him, as compared to when a nurse or stranger touches him (Massie, 1979).

As these discoveries were made, it became necessary to have instruments for assessing the longitudinal developmental significance of variations of these newborn behavioral capacities in particular children. To this end, the Brazelton (1973) Neonatal Behavior Assessment Scale is the instrument that elicits and measures the widest range of newborn behaviors. However, increasing sophistication has led specialists to recognize two significant limitations to NBAS and similar instruments such as the Graham/Rosenblith Scale (Rosenblith, 1979). First, the scales do not address the dimension of the baby's and mother's interplay; second, a newborn's degree of responsiveness in a particular area is not generally maintained from day to day, nor does it have a consistently measurable relationship to the child's later development (Sameroff, 1978). This latter finding reflects current understanding that a child's psychological development grows from a subtle and ever-shifting play of connections between environmental stimuli, biological organismic factors, infant responses, and environmental coresponses. The most important other single factor in the system is the mother, whose own actions stem from the matrix of her environment, from her character in its unconscious and conscious dimensions, and from her child's capacities for response to her (which both elicit and reciprocate maternal actions). The Scale seeks to meet the challenge of this new knowledge by functioning as an instrument that *assesses the infant's and mother's interplay;* that *can follow the evolution of dyadic behavior over a period of several months;* and that *keys on the principal newborn capacities embedded in the mutual bonding process* (Ainsworth et al., 1978; Bowlby, 1969). The infantile and maternal behaviors that compose mutual bonding—gazing, affective sharing, vocalizing, holding, touching, clinging, and physical proximity—subsequently lead to psychological interpersonal attachment (Mahler & Furer, 1968) and psychological structuring (A. Freud, 1965).

The second stream of experience which led to the development of the Scale has been our own prior research. The Early Natural History of Childhood Psychosis Project (subsequently referred to as The Project) (Massie, 1975, 1977, 1978a, 1978b). A collection was made of a series of family-made home movies of the infancies of children who subsequently developed one of the psychoses of early childhood: autism (Kanner, 1943; Ornitz & Ritvo, 1976), childhood schizophrenia (Bender, 1947), symbiotic psychosis of childhood (Mahler & Furer, 1968), or mixed patterns of illness labeled as early childhood psychosis (Rank, 1955). The movies, obtained largely from the childrens' therapists and studied together with control movies of the infancies of normal children, functioned as prospective-like data about the children's earliest life. They were examined for two classes of information: (a) the quality of reciprocal responsiveness between the mother and baby during the child's premorbid months; and (b) the documentation of the earliest symptoms of childhood psychosis, which typically appeared at about one year of age. The critical finding of the Project was that the relationship between the mother and the infant who later became ill was often disturbed as early as the first weeks of life in terms of the rhythm, reciprocity, synchronicity, and force of the aforementioned parameters of mutual bonding. In some cases the primary contribution to the aberrant interaction seemed to come from the child, in some cases from the parent.

In order to document these clinical observations, an early version of the Scale was constructed, which contained behavioral descriptions of the range and intensity of mutual responses between mother and infant as observed in the home movies of prepsychotic as well as normal infants. Further refinement of the Scale prior to field trials took place during a year of observation and piloting in the pediatric clinic at San Francisco General Hospital. This endeavor bridged the gap to the third stream of influence that has had a bearing on the development of the scale. This is the increasingly strongly felt need among child-psychiatry and pediatric specialists for an instrument with which the child-care and infant mental health practitioner can recognize aberrant parent-child interaction as early as possible. Ideally, recognition should occur in infancy in order to make possible therapeutic intervention at the earliest possible time to prevent the consolidation of severe development psychopathology.

### The Need for a Clinical Early Detection Instrument

Epidemiological surveys indicate that as many as one out of every 2,000 children may develop one of the psychoses of early childhood (Hingtgen & Bryson, 1972). Many more children develop psychophysiologic illness and character disorders such as borderline, depressive, paranoid, narcissistic, sociopathic, and obsessional personalities. Our prior research has shown how the relationship is already atypical between the baby who becomes psychotic and its mother; and clinical experience suggests that some roots of somatizing trends and other disorders also lie in disturbances of the parent-infant relationship (Greenspan et al., 1979; Roiphe, 1979). Additionally, characterologic disturbance in childhood may also be the prodromal phase of schizophrenic illness which appears in adolescence and adulthood (Cameron, 1963). Therefore it is essential from the point of view of preventive medicine that we have means to recognize these disturbed parent-child dyads. More purely neurotic difficulties, such as phobias, anxiety states, and situational reactions, are more likely to derive from experiences in the child's life subsequent to the toddler phase (A. Freud, 1965; Sperling, 1974).

Of the various psychotic syndromes of childhood, we have insufficient knowledge to specify whether there is a primary etiological defect in the child's biologic and neurologic makeup, or whether the primary fault lies in the kind of nurturing the child receives. The possible causative configurations range from the cases of children where mental illness stems entirely from a defect in a child's central nervous system, to instances where an organismically vulnerable child is also responded to with less than optimal sensitivity, or traumatically, by the parents, to cases where overwhelming parental trauma derails the psychological development of a child who has been biologically sound. In any of these instances, however, the parent-infant interaction is altered, and this becomes the window through which practitioners may identify children at risk for severe psychopathology and make their first interventions.

That early interventions in the first two years of life may succeed in arresting the progression of conditions as profound as autism has been shown in a variety of clinical reports (Call, 1963; Fraiberg et al., 1975). Nonetheless, infants in difficulty typically escape detection by their pediatricians, and only later do nursery school or kindergarten teachers note their anomalous behavior when they first venture out of their parents' homes between three and five years of age. For example, in the Project, for nine of twelve children with clear symptoms of illness appearing on their infancy films by twelve months of age, diagnosis by a professional was not made until the child had reached at least three years of age. In these nine cases the parents in eight of the families were concerned about their child's actions or lack of response at least one year before diagnosis, but could not successfully communicate their concern to pediatricians, nurses, or psychiatrists. By the time the child reaches three to five years of age, the disease process is often well established and the prognosis for successful treatment grim. This emphasizes the need for effective instruments and their use by infant-care specialists and pediatricians so that mother-infant disturbances can be identified as early as possible. Similarly, a recent review of ongoing clinical infant intervention research programs (NIMH, 1979) indicated that, although there are effective measures of infant cognitive development, there has not been an adequate armamentarium of instruments sensitive to the ongoing process of mother-infant interaction suitable for use in a clinical setting. There are at present only six measures of mother-infant interaction for use in clinical practice,[1] none of which lend themselves to rapid use in pediatric or child-care settings where early detection of

---

[1]These are the Ainsworth, Bell, and Stayton Mother-Infant Interaction Ratings; the Strange Situation Test, devised by Ainsworth et al. (1978); the Birmingham Mother-Child Interaction Measure; the Caldwell Home Inventory for Infants; the Houston Maternal Interaction Structured Situation Scales; and the Watts Mother-Child Interaction Scale.

problems must occur, nor do they focus on the actual *process* of reciprocal behavior between the mother and baby as it occurs across the
range of bonding behaviors. The Scale is designed to satisfy both
these requirements.

A number of investigators who are currently conducting research
on the process of mother-infant interaction with microanalytic studies
in a laboratory setting measure the timing and rhythm of dyadic
behaviors as they occur over seconds and fractions of seconds (Stern,
1971; Tronick et al., 1978). These careful and valuable measurements, however, are procedures that are not transferable to clinical
practice, which requires rapid appraisals without specialized equipment. To repeat, a fundamental purpose in developing the ADS
Scale has been to meet the need for simplicity and clinical practicality
in the documentation of the process of parent-infant interaction.

## Description and Use of the Attachment
## During Stress Scale

### Population

The Scale is for use with mothers and infants from birth to 18
months of age. After this age the behavior of toddlers becomes increasingly complex so that variables described by the scale are more
difficult to recognize, although they remain embedded in the maturing relationship of the mother and her child. The scale focuses on the
mother-infant relationship; but when the principal attachment figure
is not the biological mother, it is still critically important to assess the
adequacy of bonding with other parenting adults in the child's life.

### Function of the Scale

The scale attempts to quantify the reciprocal process of mother-infant
bonding by paying attention to the primary communicative and attachment behaviors available to both partners during periods when
infant and mother are undergoing a mild to moderate stress. Not only
does stress heighten and clarify the needs and responses of one member of the dyad for the other, thus making them more discernible and
ratable, but it also has important developmental significance. Normally when in distress, the infant, seeking comfort, turns to the
mother for relief and the concerned parent responds to calm the

infant. It is through experiencing such transient nontraumatic tensions and frustrations that the child gains the capacity to postpone gratification, to develop ego structures that modify instinctual demands, to differentiate intrapsychically self from other, and to individuate from the mother while maintaining stable relationships with loved ones (Mahler & Furer, 1968) who both realistically gratify and frustrate at times (Kernberg, 1975; Winnicott, 1958).

The scale therefore scrutinizes the developmentally crucial behaviors subsumed under the six basic attachment modalities of gazing, vocalizing, touching, holding, affect, and proximity. Each behavior is subdivided into component actions clinically seen in situations that arouse tension and anxiety in mother and/or infant, distributed across the scale in a range of 1 to 5 with regard to the frequency and intensity of its display during the observation period. Generally, responses at the low end of the scale (1) indicate isolation or avoidance of interaction; at the high end (5) they indicate vigorous seeking of interaction or clinging. Either extreme may be abnormal during pediatric examinations. Typical ratings lie in the middle range at 3. That is, parent and infant occasionally look at one another, occasionally "talk" with one another, and both initiate and withdraw from touching each other during the stressful period. The infant rests comfortably against its molding parent; both share an alert attentive expression appropriate to and confirming of the other's affect; and most importantly, they remain within arm's reach of each other.

When applied, the scale may serve some or all of the following functions: (1) to record the clinician's *assessment of the adequacy of maternal-infant dyadic responsiveness;* (2) to *document the need for developmental and psychological care* to prevent the crystallization of pathologic modes of social interaction and intrapsychic pathology; (3) to *document the efficacy of early intervention* efforts by registering improvement in the clinical indicators of attachment when used longitudinally during the first eighteen months of life with deviant mother-infant pairs; and (4) to *teach clinicians* by increasing their awareness of parameters of mother-infant behavior central to psychological development.

### Format of the ADS Scale

The entire scale is contained on a standard 8½ by 11-inch page. Instructions for the ADS Scale are printed on the reverse side of the rating form. The top portion of the scale quantifies the infant's behavior toward its parent; the lower portion quantifies the parent's ac-

## ADS SCALE

### THE MASSIE-CAMPBELL SCALE OF MOTHER-INFANT ATTACHMENT INDICATORS DURING STRESS

For Use During the Pediatric Examination and Other Stressful Childcare Situations

Infant's Behavior During Stress Event

| | (1) | (2) | (3) | (4) | (5) | X |
|---|---|---|---|---|---|---|
| GAZING | $\frac{1}{1}$ Always looks away from mother's face. | $\frac{2}{1}$ Rarely searches out mother's face. Fleeting looks at mother's face. | $\frac{3}{1}$ Occasionally looks at mother's face. | $\frac{4}{1}$ Frequently long & short gazing at mother's face. | $\frac{5}{1}$ Rivets gaze on mother's face for long periods. | $\frac{6}{1}$ Behavior not observed. |
| VOCALIZING | $\frac{1}{2}$ Quiet. Never vocalizing. | $\frac{2}{2}$ Rarely vocalizing or whimpering. | $\frac{3}{2}$ Occasionally vocalizing or mild crying. | $\frac{4}{2}$ Frequently vocalizing or intense crying. | $\frac{5}{2}$ Uncontrollable, intense crying much of time. | $\frac{6}{2}$ Behavior not observed. |
| TOUCHING (a) | $\frac{1}{3}$ Never touches or reaches toward mother. | $\frac{2}{3}$ Rarely touches mother. | $\frac{3}{3}$ Occasionally touches mother. | $\frac{4}{3}$ Frequently reaches toward & touches mother. | $\frac{5}{3}$ When close, always touching mother. | $\frac{6}{3}$ Behavior not observed. |
| (b) | $\frac{1}{4}$ Always pulls away from mother's touch. | $\frac{2}{4}$ Frequently pulls away from her touch. | $\frac{3}{4}$ Occasionally pulls away from her touch. | $\frac{4}{4}$ Rarely pulls away from her touch. | $\frac{5}{4}$ Never pulls away from her touch. | $\frac{6}{4}$ Behavior not observed. |
| HOLDING | $\frac{1}{5}$ Violently resists holding; always arches away from mother. | $\frac{2}{5}$ Does not relax in mother's arms. Frequently pulls away. | $\frac{3}{5}$ Rests in mother's arms and against her shoulder. Occasionally pulls away. | $\frac{4}{5}$ Body molds to mother's. Rarely pulls away. | $\frac{5}{5}$ Actively turns & arches body toward mother's. Clings strongly. Never pulls away. | $\frac{6}{5}$ Behavior not observed. |
| AFFECT | $\frac{1}{6}$ Always intensely anguished & fearful. | $\frac{2}{6}$ Frequently irritable, fearful or apathetic. | $\frac{3}{6}$ Intermittent moderate anxiety and/or pleasure; or unclear. | $\frac{4}{6}$ Rare tension; largely smiling. | $\frac{5}{6}$ Always smiling. | $\frac{6}{6}$ Behavior not observed. |
| PROXIMITY | $\frac{1}{7}$ Never follows mother bodily or with eyes; goes to far corner or out of room. | $\frac{2}{7}$ Rarely follows mother bodily or with eyes; often at far corner of room from mother. | $\frac{3}{7}$ Intermittently follows mother bodily or with eyes. | $\frac{4}{7}$ Frequently follows mother bodily or with eyes. | $\frac{5}{7}$ Always follows mother bodily or with eyes. | $\frac{6}{7}$ Behavior not observed. |

Mother's Response to Infant's Stress

| | (1) | (2) | (3) | (4) | (5) | X |
|---|---|---|---|---|---|---|
| GAZING | $\frac{1}{8}$ Always looks away from child's face. | $\frac{2}{8}$ Rarely looks at child's face. Fleeting looks at child's face. | $\frac{3}{8}$ Occasionally looks at child's face. | $\frac{4}{8}$ Frequently long & short gazing at child's face. | $\frac{5}{8}$ Rivets gaze on child's face for long periods. | $\frac{6}{8}$ Behavior not observed. |
| VOCALIZING | $\frac{1}{9}$ Quiet. Never vocalizing. | $\frac{2}{9}$ Rare words, cooing or murmuring. | $\frac{3}{9}$ Occasionally vocalizing to child. | $\frac{4}{9}$ Frequently speaks, murmurs, coos. | $\frac{5}{9}$ Intense vocalizations throughout exam. | $\frac{6}{9}$ Behavior not observed. |
| TOUCHING (a) | $\frac{1}{10}$ Never touches or reaches toward child. | $\frac{2}{10}$ Rarely touches child. | $\frac{3}{10}$ Occasionally touches child. | $\frac{4}{10}$ Frequently reaches toward & touches child. | $\frac{5}{10}$ When close, always touching child. | $\frac{6}{10}$ Behavior not observed. |
| (b) | $\frac{1}{11}$ Always pulls away from his touch. | $\frac{2}{11}$ Frequently pulls away from his touch. | $\frac{3}{11}$ Occasionally pulls away from his touch. | $\frac{4}{11}$ Rarely pulls away from his touch. | $\frac{5}{11}$ Never pulls away from his touch. | $\frac{6}{11}$ Behavior not observed. |
| HOLDING | $\frac{1}{12}$ Pushes upset child away, or holds away from body. | $\frac{2}{12}$ Holds child stiffly & awkwardly. Not relaxed. | $\frac{3}{12}$ Supports child relaxedly against her chest or shoulder briefly. | $\frac{4}{12}$ Body molds to child & maintains contact until child quiets. | $\frac{5}{12}$ Body inclines toward child, followed by prolonged holding with molding. | $\frac{6}{12}$ Behavior not observed. |
| AFFECT | $\frac{1}{13}$ Always intensely anguished & fearful. | $\frac{2}{13}$ Frequently irritable, fearful or apathetic. | $\frac{3}{13}$ Intermittent moderate anxiety and/or pleasure; or unclear. | $\frac{4}{13}$ Rare tension; largely smiling. | $\frac{5}{13}$ Always smiling. | $\frac{6}{13}$ Behavior not observed. |
| PROXIMITY | $\frac{1}{14}$ Leaves examining room. | $\frac{2}{14}$ Frequently out of reach of child; or at far corner of room from child. | $\frac{3}{14}$ Intermittent standing or seated within arm's reach of child. | $\frac{4}{14}$ Frequently in physical contact with child. | $\frac{5}{14}$ Always in physical contact with child. | $\frac{6}{14}$ Behavior not observed. |

© 1977 Henry N. Massie, M.D., and B. Kay Campbell, Ph.D.

*261*

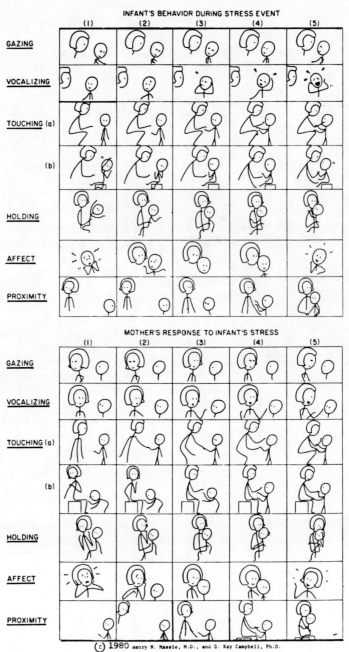

Illustrative drawings of mother-infant behaviors described by the ADS Scale.

tions; and at the bottom are spaces to record demographic and historical information. A page of drawings also translates to the printed page the behaviors we have studied.

### Setting of the Observation and Rating

The Scale has been developed largely in the context of the pediatric clinic during well-baby physical examinations, a mildly stressful experience for mother and child. The context provides the only consistent opportunity that child-care specialists have for assessing the quality of the mother-infant relationship—an assessment which we believe should be a routine component of pediatric care.

The Scale may also be applied in other settings where a mild stress occurs to assess parent-infant reciprocity. Such settings may be naturally occurring events in which some tension predictably occurs, such as dressing, bathing, playing, and family mealtimes. A typical naturally occurring stress is the moment of mother-infant separation or reunion that a child-care worker may observe at a daycare center. The investigator may also wish to create a structured and standardized brief mother-infant separation and reunion experience to rate with the Scale as Ainsworth has done with the Strange Situation Test (Ainsworth et al., 1978). With such a paradigm, the Scale rating could document the social interactions occurring during the leave-taking and during reunion between mother and baby. In any case the usefulness of the Scale is enhanced by its repeated application in the same setting.

### Equipment and Space Required

The only equipment required is a pen or pencil with which to mark the observations. The pediatric examination room should be large enough to accommodate mother, baby, and pediatrician. If the pediatrician is not making the Scale observations, room for an additional observer is needed. There must be sufficient room for the mother to be able to sit next to her infant or hold her infant. A fresh copy of the Scale should be used for each rating so that the judgment of the rater is not affected by markings of previous ratings given the mother-infant pair.

Scale Instructions

# INTRODUCTION

The Attachment Indicators During Stress Scale is to be used with infants from birth to 18 months of age to detect aberrant mother-infant responsiveness in stressful situations. The Scale quantifies the reciprocal process of mother-infant attachment while the infant is under the stress of an ordinary physical examination. The Scale can also be used in other situations which produce tension in mother and baby. When stressed, infants normatively seek out their mothers; mothers normatively seek out their infants when they perceive them to be in danger or suffering. Such interactions fall within the general category of attachment behaviors. The Scale includes six basic attachment modalities: gazing, vocalizing, touching, and holding, affect and proximity. These modalities are subdivided into component behaviors and correspond to mother and infant responses clinically seen in stressful situations which arouse tension and anxiety in mother and/or infant. The responses in each attachment modality are graded from 1 to 5 to indicate the increasing intensity of mother-infant involvement that may occur during a stress episode. Generally, behavior at the low end of the Scale (1) indicates abnormal isolation or avoidance of attachment, and responses at the high end (5) indicate abnormally anxious attachment behavior or clinging. The top half of the single-page Scale quantifies the infant's behavior with its mother, and the bottom half quantifies the mother's behavior with her infant during the stressful situation.

# APPLICATIONS

The ADS Scale is for use during the pediatric examination as well as other situations where a relatively standardized stress occurs for parents and babies. For example, it can be used by mental health or childcare workers to assess mother-infant attachment at the moment of reunion following the stress of a brief separation between mother and child. In whatever setting it is used it may serve some or all of the following functions:

1) To record the clinician's assessment of the adequacy of maternal infant dyadic responsiveness.

2) To document the need for developmental and psychological care to prevent the crystallization of pathological modes of social interaction.

3) To document the efficacy of early intervention efforts by registering improvement in the clinical indicators of attachment when used longitudinally during the first 18 months of life with deviant mother-infant pairs.

4) To teach by heightening the clinician's awareness of parameters of mother-infant interaction central to psychological development.

# INSTRUCTIONS FOR ADMINISTRATION AND SCORING

The clinician conducting the examination or an independent observer can administer the ADS Scale. Generally, the mother should not be alerted to the details of the observation so that she does not modify her usual style; and for the same reason the examiner should not suggest to the mother that she either hold the baby or place the baby on the examining table, but instead leave the decision with the mother.

To use the Scale, observe the interaction between mother and infant WHILE the infant is being physically examined (the *stress episode*) and IMMEDIATELY AFTERWARD (the *reunion and recovery episode*). In many pediatric examinations the final phase is the inspection of the head, eyes, ears, nose and throat. This usually takes about 3 minutes and is often the most difficult for mother and infant. The period immediately following this (about 3 minutes) is the time when mother and infant reunite and tension subsides. Similarly, in non-pediatric settings there is a corresponding rise and fall of tension around a stressful event. Assessment is made by focusing on the period of most heightened stress (the final 3 minutes of the physical examination) and the period of tension decline (the first 3 minutes of the recovery phase). IMMEDIATELY AFTER THE OBSERVATION OF THE RECOVERY EPISODE circle the behavior description that best fits the mother's and infant's response in each attachment modality during both stress and recovery episodes. If a particular attachment modality, such as holding, has not occurred circle "not observed" so that an entry is made in every category.

264

## OPERATIONAL DEFINITIONS

Holding: the mutually reciprocated posturing of the infant and mother while the infant is supported in the arms of the mother.

Gazing: the eye-to-face contact within a dyad and the maintenance of this contact.

Vocalizing: the making of vocal sounds for the benefit of the partner in the mother-infant dyad. The infant's crying is considered a vocal signal of dismay during stress which alerts the mother to its tension.

Touching (a): the making of skin-to-skin contact initiated by either the mother or the infant for play or attention not physical support.

Touching (b): the withdrawal from skin-to-skin contact initiated by either the mother or the infant.

Affect: the facial expressions signaling emotional states. A bland expression is considered typical of the individual under stress and is appropriate.

Proximity: the state of being near, close to, or beside another. In the context of the ADS Scale it refers to the infant maintaining either physical or visual contact with the mother, and to the mother maintaining physical contact or being immediately accessible to her infant.

Rarely: the behavior occurs once in a while, or seldom; it doesn't happen often during the observation period.

Occasionally: the behavior occurs from time to time, now and then during the observation period.

Frequently: the behavior happens often but not all the time during the observation period.

## INTERPRETATION OF SCORING

Normal behaviors will usually rate at 3 and 4. When an infant or a mother rates at 1 or 2 it suggests that the infant or mother may be either avoiding contact or not responding to the other's display of tension or attempts at attachment. When there are scores of 5 it should raise concern that there is an over-anxious intense attachment or an unusually strong reaction to stress. Further, in dyads where one member rates at 1 or 2 and the other at 5, there is a dissynchrony of interaction which may also have pathological significance. To derive a single or "correct" score is *not* the proper use of the Scale. The most productive way to interpret the ratings is to use the attachment indicators as a guide to the adequacy of interaction in a given mother-infant pair. Studies indicate that deviant attachment is associated with subsequent psychomotor developmental delays, pathological intrapsychic management of tension and aggression, and the inability to postpone gratification—all with their attendant behavioral disturbances. When behaviors of 1, 2, or 5 occur in 2 successive episodes, there should be a diagnostic workup, for, once established, unhealthy patterns of mother-infant interaction show little change without therapeutic intervention. The exception occurs with some very young or premature infants who show a normal dampened responsiveness. They may rate 2 for gazing, vocalizing, touching (a), and proximity in the first weeks of life. Mother-infant affect at 5 at any age is not necessarily clinging but is aberrant.

## VARIABLES

Relatively standardized stress situations may be affected by several variables. An infant's ability to tolerate tension or respond to comforting may be affected, for example, by concurrent illness or hunger. Likewise, a mother's capacities may be affected by concurrent disturbances in her life. History taking should elicit this; and the ADS Scale can then assist in assessing the capacity of the mother and infant to compensate for additional stress, or their liability for decompensation and the traumatic behaviors that follow. Additionally, a disturbing examining situation or other unusual circumstances can intensify the stress of customary events. If there are unusual occurrences when the rating takes place explain briefly in the space provided at the bottom of the Scale.

Fathers accompany infants less frequently than mothers, but the ADS Scale can be appropriately used to assess father-infant interaction. When infants are older than 18 months their behaviors have become so increasingly complex that the ADS Scale is less useful.

### Operational Definitions of the ADS Scale Attachment Behaviors

It is important that users of the Scale share clear and unambiguous definitions of each of the behaviors to be observed, as follows:

*Gazing:*   the eye-to-face contact within a dyad and the maintenance of this contact.

*Holding:*   the mutually reciprocated posturing of the infant and mother while the infant is supported in the arms of the mother.

*Vocalizing:*   the making of vocal sounds for the benefit of the partner in the parent-infant dyad. The infant's crying is considered a signal of dismay during stress, which alerts the parent to its tension.

*Touching (a):*   Skin-to-skin contact initiated by either parent or infant for play or affection, not for physical support.

*Touching (b):*   the withdrawal from skin-to-skin contact initiated by either parent or infant. (Touching (a) and (b) does not refer to contact in the service of holding, clinging, or body support. Rather it refers to playful grooming, affectionate, communicative, or other touching that may be expressed, for example, by fingers, hands, feet, toes, or facial nuzzling.)

*Affect:*   the facial expressions signaling emotional states. An unclear, slightly anxious, alert, attentive, or bland expression is considered typical of the individual under stress and is appropriate.

*Proximity:*   the state of being near, close to, or beside another. In the context of the ADS Scale, it refers to the infant's maintaining either physical or visual contact with the parent, and to the parent's maintaining physical contact or being immediately accessible to the infant.

*Rarely:*   the behavior occurs once in a while; it doesn't happen often during the observation period.

*Occasionally:* the behavior occurs from time to time, now and then during the observation period.

*Frequently:* the behavior happens often but not all the time during the observation period.

*Always:* the behavior constantly occurs during the observational period.

*Never:* the behavior does not occur during the observation period.

*Behavior Not Observed:* this category is reserved for those occasions when the observer was not able to observe specific behaviors in question due to an awkward or obstructed range of vision or when a behavior did not take place (for example, if a mother never held her baby).

### Instructions for Administration and Scoring

Either the clinician conducting the infant's physical examination or an observer can administer the Scale. The clinician should, as in all clinical settings, assist parent and infant to feel as relaxed and free to engage with each other as the situation permits. To facilitate this, the physician may choose to begin the interview by reviewing the infant's history since the previous visit and by asking for the demographic information and social history that is requested at the bottom of the scale if it is not already available. The examiner should not alert the parent to the details of the ADS Scale observations so that the mother does not modify her usual style. For the same reason the examiner should not suggest to the mother that she either hold or place the baby on the examining table, but should leave the decision with her, since the mother's choice in this matter is potentially an indicator of how she handles the modes of physical proximity and holding with her child.

To use the scale, observe the interaction between parent and infant *while* the infant is being physically examined *(the stress period)* and *immediately afterward (the reunion and recovery period).* In many pediatric examinations, the final phase is the inspection of the head, eyes, ears, nose, and throat. This usually takes about three minutes and is often the most difficult for parent and infant. The period immediately following (about three minutes) is the time when parent and infant are reunited and tension subsides. Similarly, in nonpediatric settings, there is a corresponding rise and fall of tension around a stressful event.

Assessment is made by focusing on the period of most heightened stress (the final three minutes of the physical examination) and the period of tension decline (the first three minutes of the recovery phase). *Immediately after the observation of the recovery episode,* circle the behavioral description that best fits the infant's and parent's response in each attachment modality during the entire observation period (the stress and recovery episodes). If a particular behavior, such as holding, has not occurred during the observation period, circle "not observed." It is important that an entry is made for each of the seven behaviors.

### Interpretation of Scoring

Normal behaviors will usually be rated 3 and 4. Lower ratings suggest that the infant or parent may either be avoiding contact, or not responding to the other's display of tension or attempts at attachment. Scores of 5 should raise concern that there may be overanxious and intense attachment, or an unusually strong reaction to stress on the part of mother, child, or both. In dyads where one member rates at 1 or 2 and the other at 5, there is a dissynchrony of interaction which may also have pathological significance. The most productive way to interpret the ratings are as descriptive guides to the adequacy of interaction within a parent-infant dyad. The scale is not designed to produce a single "correct" score.

When two or more behaviors have been rated at 1, 2, and/or 5 on at least two successive visits, empirical clinical judgment would indicate that there should be a diagnostic evaluation, including a social and psychiatric history of both parents and infant. It appears that once unhealthy patterns of social behavior are established they become integrated into overall interactional styles that are shared between dyadic partners, recur on repeated evaluations, and show little change without therapeutic intervention. In our experience, when aberrant interactional patterns are serially observed, the child may be at risk for impaired psychological development.

There are exceptions to this outline of typical response. Some very young or premature infants may show social behaviors that are considerably subdued. They have a normal dampened responsiveness and may receive low ratings in gazing, touching (a), vocalizing, and proximity in the first weeks of life. Further clinical study of the case, however, would clarify the reason for the low ratings, and possibly guide supportive counselling for parents who felt frustrated that their involvement with their baby was not being rewarded by greater responsiveness from the child. In addition, mother or infant affect rated at 5 at any age is not necessarily indicative of a clinging mother. Alternatively, it may also bespeak denial of less happy feelings, and is nonetheless aberrant. A persistent smile (5) in the face of stress is an abnormal absence of signaling of tension indicative of a difficulty in the parent's or infant's expression of anxiety. It may be an outgrowth of a failure of interpersonal connectedness between partners in the dyad; it may also reflect a child's early identification with a parent who has a particularly noncommunicative affective style.

Although the scale primarily assists in characterizing patterns of parent-infant interaction, it may also be a principal tool in the diagnosis of three of the four major psychiatric conditions of the first eighteen months of life. These are autism (and the phenomenologically very similar deprivation syndrome), infantile depression, and symbiotic psychosis of childhood. Infantile eating disturbances, the fourth infant psychiatric condition, are not directly visualizable with routine use of the Scale. Nonetheless, when one case of infantile anorexia was studied closely (Massie, 1980), there appeared a marked skewing of the responses of both child and mother toward angry and avoidant behaviors (1's and 2's).

*Autism:*   When an autistic syndrome exists, the pathology is clearly evident in routine use of the Scale. In our experience the infant consistently rates at the avoidant level of 1 to 2. The mother's behavior might range from anxious or vigorous attempts to elicit responses from her child (4 and 5) to frustrated or resigned withdrawal from her child (1 and 2).

*Infantile Depressions:*   These conditions are usually associated with loss of the mothering figure in the first year of life. (Bowlby, 1951; Spitz & Wolf, 1946), whether by mother's physical absence, or secondary to her own depression, severe preoccupation, or self-involvement. Clinically depressed infants appear emotionally withdrawn, isolated, and fail to develop loving ties with other people. On the Scale they may show apathetic responses (ratings of 1 and 2) though not necessarily ratings of 1 for touching (b) or holding, which are found to reflect the admixture of willful avoidance exhibited by some autistic children. When the mother is physically present but emotionally unavailable due to her own depression or difficulties, her interaction parallels the depressed infant's in terms of low ratings and unresponsiveness. In the closely related infantile depressions which derive from a child's identification with a depressed mother and her depressed facies, the mother's apathetic actions with her child are reflected in the baby's responses (Adelson & Fraiberg, 1977), and both mother and infant receive low Scale scores.

*Symbiotic Psychosis of Childhood:*    This syndrome is diagnosed by the toddler's responding to the experience or threat of separation from the mother with severe behavioral regression, a display of aggression and anxiety, and loss of most or all of the independent functioning it has achieved. Interactional components are easier to determine from the maternal side. A parent may have particular needs, arising from her own life history, to rigidly control her infant out of a personal drive for dominance, or from hostility toward that child. She may guard against expressing her hostility by overanxious and close attachment. A mother may also have a pressing need to establish a close union with her infant so that she herself experiences the feeling of being nurtured and loved by the baby. In any event, the outcome for the child is severely impaired ego development associated with inadequate self-object differentiation. In some cases a significant organic condition may contribute to the child's impaired ego development, which makes the separation-individuation process more perilous and optimal parental auxilliary ego functioning more essential for the child. Typically, multiple scale ratings of 5 are found, indicative of an overly intense involvement between mother and child. In situations where the parent has a hostile need to control the baby and experiences difficulty nurturing, there may also appear low ratings for touching (b), holding, and affect on the parent's part.

Users should note that many dyads will show non-normative Scale ratings in mildly stressful situations and most of these children will not go on to develop psychotic level psychopathology. For example, difficulty in the separation-individuation process—appearing as unusually strong clinging or physical closeness between mother and child, or a parent's mistrust of the child's spending time with others—may perhaps lead to school phobias, learning inhibitions, and psychophysiological gastrointestinal, respiratory, allergic, and somatic disorders. Such abnormal bonding patterns are not obligatorily related to psychosis in most instances, and further longitudinal research is needed to establish possible connections between parent-infant interactional configurations and these disturbances.

*Additional Considerations and Examiner Training*

The stress of the pediatric examination is rarely intense, since clinicians are most often able to complete a physical examination without alarming their young patients. However, concurrent family upset or illness or hunger in the child may affect the ratings. History-taking and the physical examination should elicit this. The Scale may then assist in assessing the capacity of the parent and infant to compensate for additional stress, or their liability for decompensation and the traumatic behaviors that follow. But in general, reactions to the same stress should be assessed over time in order to identify the pattern of interaction a particular parent-infant pair establish between themselves.

The Scale should be administered by infant-development and child-care professionals familiar with normal and abnormal patterns of social interaction and infant maturational and developmental pathways. Supervised training and practice sessions in the administration of the Scale are strongly recommended. Training should include opportunities to observe live or taped healthy parent-infant dyads interacting during standard stress situations, allowing students repeated opportunities to view the various behaviors to be rated and to compare their ratings with those of experienced observers. The operational definitions of the behavior should be reviewed and compared as they appear in various levels of intensity. Opportunities should also be provided to rate filmed or videotaped examinations of parent-infant pairs at serious risk, showing dissynchronous behaviors between parent and infant or behaviors at the extremes of the rating scale for both members of the pair. Comparisons of these parents and infants at risk with those receiving normal ratings are necessary to illuminate the behavioral differences. Finally, time should be allotted to discuss the interpretation of the Scale rating. Periodic retraining sessions with peer-group consultation minimize administrator distortions.

## Statistical Studies

*Concurrent and Predictive Validity*

The Scale is a relatively new instrument. Whereas clinical experience documents its effectiveness in identifying current difficulties within a given mother-infant relationship, there are still insufficient data to allow a statement about the scale's predictive validity with regard to future pathology. The scale has been useful in showing that early interactional patterns, once established, do persist over time, but it is not yet possible to discuss the overall implications of such persistent behavior when seen in a large number of cases. A small pilot group of cases we have followed from birth to three-and-a-half years of age does provide an initial concrete indication of the predictive usefulness of the scale. In this study, six families wherein Scale behavior in the first weeks of life indicated poor bonding (low ratings), and seven families wherein the mother-infant interaction in the first weeks of life was unremarkable by Scale ratings, were restudied at three-and-a-half years. An independent clinician who did not know about their original grouping found that the originally poorly bonding children were now showing a trend to less happy affect, less spontaneity, less concentration on tasks, and sparser communication and reciprocity with examiner and parent than the normally attaching group. In addition, caution is important when considering the predictive value of consistency and stability of maternal behavior. A child must be able to anticipate parental behaviors in the process of learning to identify and control its own actions. However, a parent whose behavior is consistent but aberrant may be equally pathogenic as one whose behavior is unpredictable. When studying action patterns, it is not enough to describe consistency or unpredictability; one must discuss the particular structure of the pattern, and under which circumstances and which conditions. The Scale provides a view of interpersonal behavior under stress that enables comparisons of stress-related behaviors over time. It is important that the clinician exercise judgment in interpreting and predicting future behavior based upon Scale ratings.

### Interrater Reliability

When careful training is given to users of the scale, there is good agreement among observers of episodes of mother-infant behavior. To demonstrate this, four reliability studies have been conducted using formulas developed by Willemson (1977) for analyses of data generated by more than one pair of judges observing mother-infant interaction. Consensual agreement across fourteen descriptive categories ranged from 0.34 to 0.80; agreement within one scale point ranged from 0.83 to 0.99.

*Standardization—The Normative Sample*

The standardizing sample was drawn from the Early Periodic Screening, Diagnosis and Treatment Program (1969) which was jointly conducted by the Michigan Departments of Public Health and of Mental Health.[2] Infants were brought to the EPSDT Programs by their mothers for routine health care, and the group included both sick and well babies. Over a five-month period the Scale was administered to 228 mother-infant pairs. Forty pairs were excluded because of infant age and/or missing data (for instance, sex of infant), but general sample characteristics were based on the total sample of 228 pairs. This group represented 1.5 percent of the infants eighteen months and younger in the five Michigan counties where the scale was used. Communities participating in the study ranged from a population of close to 200,000 to rural towns with approximately 30,000 inhabitants (U.S. Dept. of Commerce, 1977).

Participation was voluntary, and parental consent was secured before Scale assessments were performed. Clinicians introduced the test by explaining they were interested in "assessing the baby's sociability" as part of their routine physical examinations. No parental refusals were reported.

The infants tested ranged in age from birth to eighteen months, but because only a small number of infants tested were over twelve months of age, the final normative tables were based on information from infants tested in their first year of life. Girls and boys were placed in separate groups; the groups were divided into four age periods: 1–90 days, 91–180 days, 181–270 days, and 271–360 days. First and later-born infants were included in the sample and were equally distributed across the research population (Table 1). Mothers in the sample were from fourteen to forty-one years of age, with an average age of twenty-five years. Approximately a third of the mothers were single parents.

Among the families studied 91 percent had a yearly income of $10,000 or less, making the sample representative of low-income families who would be served by government-subsidized medical clinics.

---

[2]The data was gathered under the supervision of Richard Spates, Ph,D., Director, Evaluation, Design, and Analysis Division, Budget and Evaluation System, State of Michigan Department of Mental Health; Betty Tableman, Infant Mental Health Director, Department of Mental Health, State of Michigan; and Mary K. Peterson, R.N., Infant Mental Health Specialist, Department of Mental Health, State of Michigan.

**TABLE 1** *Sample by age and sex*

| Age periods | Male infants | Female infants | Total |
|---|---|---|---|
| 1– 90 days | 33 | 45 | 78 |
| 91–180 days | 26 | 25 | 51 |
| 181–270 days | 16 | 17 | 33 |
| 271–360 days | 14 | 12 | 26 |
| Total Sample | 89 | 99 | 188 |

$x^2 = 1.48$, df $= 3$, p n.s.

An analysis showed that variations for each attachment category by infant sex and age were statistically not significant. It is therefore assumed that the ratings on the Scale are not affected by the age or sex of the infant in the mother-infant pair under assessment. Data generated by the 5-point Scale is negatively skewed and leptokurtic (that is, the shape of the distribution tends to be more peaked than a normal curve). This is a function of the scale's design and one that makes it clinically useful but statistically awkward. When one standard deviation was added or subtracted from the mean, the range in some cases extended to over 5.00 (touching [b], boys, age 181–270 days) and to just below 2.00 (vocalizing, mothers of boys, age 181–270 days). This suggests that caution should be used in making judgments based on the ratings. No "at risk" designation should be applied unless there have been two or more ratings at or below 2 or at 5 for either mother and/or infant on two successive visits; and serial episodes generating aberrant values must be augmented by clinical review and evaluation of the families.

An interesting finding was that within the field of nursing, more highly trained clinicians rate samples of mother-infant intereaction during the pediatric examination higher on the Scale than their less-trained counterparts. In this regard, health screening of children is a primary component of the advanced training and role of the pediatric nurse clinician. As a function of their education, these nurses may be more likely to tolerate diversity within the patients, thereby being less critical of variations in behavior. Conversely, the role of the lesser trained nurse is more closely aligned with the "cure" functions performed by physicians (Christensen et al., 1979), with a focus more on parameters of pathology and restoration of behavior to standard norms. The differences on the Scale ratings of these pro-

274

fessional groups could be attributed to such biases and bears further investigation.

*Abnormal Ratings: Physically Ill Infants:* Within the sample of 228 mother-infant pairs, thirty infants were physically sick when they received Scale ratings. Based upon this small number, it appears there may be a difference between the sexes in behavior presented when physically sick. Among the sick girls 63 percent were rated abnormally, the majority of their Scale ratings being 1 and 2, that is, withdrawing from social interaction with their mothers. Only 31 percent of the sick boys tended to rate abnormally, and the majority of those ratings were 5, suggesting that the boys were more demanding of maternal social involvement when they were not feeling well. Illnesses included respiratory and ear infections, growth disturbances, and cardiovascular and skin disorders.

*Abnormal Ratings: Physically Well Infants:* Abnormal Scale ratings appeared for physically healthy infants and their mothers in fifty-eight of the 228 pairs in the sample. That is, 25 percent of the mother-infant pairs received multiple scores of 1, 2, or 5 in a single (non-serial) examination. These findings are similar to figures from an urban city hospital in California where 20 percent of 127 mother-infant pairs in the well-baby clinic received multiple scores of 1, 2, or 5 on a single Scale rating (Campbell, 1977). That same 20 percent were found to have the same ratings on at least one subsequent visit. If the Scale does function as a preliminary screener, alerting the clinician to infants at risk for the subsequent development of psychopathology, the proportion of children so selected should be somewhat higher than the number that eventually suffer from consolidated psychiatric illness. It is instructive, therefore, to observe that, in the United States, out of 157 million outpatient visits to physicians by children under 15 years of age (HEW, 1975), 12 percent were for psychiatric conditions. And a survey (MacFarlane et al., 1962) of severe behavior problems of children—soiling, enuresis, tics, hyperactivity, speech disorders, antisocial behavior, and fearful or dependent qualities— indicated that 9 percent of children under fifteen years of age will exhibit one or more of these problems. In the same survey approximately double this number exhibited difficulties of a more minor and less pathognomonic degree.

The standardization studies to date are incomplete, and the numbers of mother-infant pairs rated at each age group are modest.

## TABLE 2 ADS scale norms
### Means and standard deviations by sex and age

| Age in days | Infants | | | | | | | | | | | | | |
|---|---|---|---|---|---|---|---|---|---|---|---|---|---|---|
| | Gazing | | Vocalizing | | Touch A | | Touch B | | Holding | | Affect | | Proximity | |
| | $M^1$ | $S.D.^2$ | M | S.D. | M | S.D. | M | S.D. | M | S.D. | M | S.D. | M | S.D. |
| **Boys** | | | | | | | | | | | | | | |
| 1– 90 | 3.39 | .74 | 3.12 | .76 | 3.37 | .59 | 3.69 | .63 | 3.64 | .58 | 3.15 | .63 | 3.30 | .66 |
| 91–180 | 3.50 | .76 | 3.19 | .74 | 3.30 | 1.01 | 3.82 | .57 | 3.64 | .56 | 3.65 | .74 | 3.46 | .64 |
| 181–270 | 3.68 | .79 | 3.35 | 1.00 | 3.73 | .96 | 3.66 | .61 | 3.64 | .74 | 3.53 | .99 | 3.43 | .72 |
| 271–360 | 3.57 | .85 | 3.33 | 1.04 | 3.80 | .67 | 4.26 | .79 | 3.69 | .75 | 3.13 | 1.18 | 3.13 | .63 |
| **Girls** | | | | | | | | | | | | | | |
| 1– 90 | 3.17 | .86 | 3.17 | .71 | 3.02 | .73 | 3.66 | .47 | 3.66 | .57 | 2.95 | .63 | 3.07 | .60 |
| 91–180 | 3.48 | .65 | 3.40 | .50 | 3.62 | 1.09 | 3.87 | .74 | 3.64 | .70 | 3.40 | .76 | 3.40 | .50 |
| 181–270 | 3.47 | .62 | 3.58 | .93 | 3.41 | .71 | 4.05 | .55 | 3.76 | .66 | 3.41 | 1.06 | 3.58 | .87 |
| 271–360 | 3.33 | .98 | 3.41 | .79 | 3.83 | .71 | 3.75 | 1.05 | 3.58 | .79 | 2.83 | .57 | 3.66 | .65 |
| **Mothers of boys** | | | | | | | | | | | | | | |
| 1– 90 | 3.64 | .58 | 3.36 | .67 | 3.57 | .75 | 3.93 | .51 | 3.41 | .84 | 3.45 | .50 | 3.50 | .64 |
| 91–180 | 3.80 | .57 | 3.04 | .84 | 3.28 | .93 | 3.95 | .57 | 3.68 | .69 | 3.56 | .71 | 3.36 | .86 |
| 181–270 | 3.73 | .59 | 3.00 | 1.15 | 3.30 | .85 | 3.75 | .62 | 3.50 | .63 | 3.56 | .51 | 3.37 | .61 |
| 271–360 | 3.86 | .51 | 3.46 | .83 | 3.80 | .67 | 4.14 | .66 | 3.53 | .66 | 3.93 | .45 | 3.80 | .56 |
| **Mothers of girls** | | | | | | | | | | | | | | |
| 1– 90 | 3.56 | .68 | 3.20 | .78 | 3.46 | .75 | 3.78 | .62 | 3.65 | .62 | 3.60 | .57 | 3.52 | .65 |
| 91–180 | 3.76 | .51 | 3.44 | .86 | 3.42 | .94 | 3.95 | .84 | 3.56 | .91 | 3.57 | .57 | 3.53 | .64 |
| 181–270 | 3.70 | .68 | 3.38 | .69 | 3.70 | .58 | 4.00 | .51 | 3.41 | .71 | 3.64 | .49 | 3.58 | .71 |
| 271–360 | 3.91 | .51 | 3.08 | .99 | 4.00 | .60 | 4.08 | .66 | 3.75 | .62 | 3.58 | .66 | 3.83 | .83 |

[1]M = mean rating assigned each age group for the variable
[2]S.D. = standard deviation of the mean

Nonetheless, the normative tables that have been prepared showing the means and standard deviations of Scale ratings for infants in sex and age should be of use to clinicians and researchers. So, too, should the clinical assumptions and experiences from which the scale itself is constructed. With further use of the instrument in the future, the theoretical and empirical bases of the scale may be more precisely shown to be predictive of some of the psychiatric disturbances that occur in older children and adults.

## CASE EXAMPLES

### Bill

From birth the child regurgitated his feedings, and at one month was diagnosed as having pyloric stenosis. Shortly thereafter he was hospitalized for successful surgery, but his recuperation kept him in the hospital until his third month of life. Bill's parents, both mature and dependable, visited regularly, and his mother participated in his feedings. Scale ratings were obtained a month after discharge during a routine examination in the pediatric clinic. Bill rated at 2 for gazing, vocalizing, affect, and proximity; he scored 1 for touching (a) and 3 for touching (b) and holding. Descriptively, Bill rarely vocalized. He looked irritable and fearful. He never reached toward his mother to touch her and occasionally pulled away from her. The mother, on her part, rated consistently at 3 in all categories: she occasionally looked at Bill's face, talked to him and touched him. She stayed within arm's reach throughout the examination. She occasionally pulled away from his touch but more often initiated touches and appeared relaxed as she held him against her. Her facial expression was attentive, neither smiling nor frowning excessively.

These ratings demonstrate that, although Bill was not an avoidant child, his social behaviors were less than those of a normal child. His mother was socially engaging with him. Interpretation of these behaviors suggested that the child's separations from his parents as well as the trauma of surgery and its interference with sensorimotor contact with both his parents and his environment had interfered with Bill's normal attachment to his mother as well as with adaptation to the environment. The mother, on her part, was loving of her son but perplexed about how active to be with him. On the basis of these observations the pediatrician suggested to the mother the need and appropriateness for her to augment her activities with her baby, and encouraged her tolerance of his unusually muted responses to her overtures. After some weeks a repeat Scale examination indicated a reciprocal movement in the direction of greater involvement on the part of both mother and infant, reflecting mutually appropriate responses under stress.

## Michael

Michael's family showed more serious maladaptive interaction and was far more difficult for pediatricians and psychotherapists to intervene with successfully. The unmarried mother first appeared in the well-baby clinic when Michael was three months old. A nurse quickly noted how the mother left her baby at times unattended on the examining table even when there was no one else in the room. Scale ratings during the pediatric examination gave Michael ratings of 1 in gazing, vocalizing, touching (a), and affect. He was given ratings of 2 in touching (b), holding, and proximity. The mother showed equally withdrawing and avoidant behaviors: she received ratings of 1 in vocalizing, holding, proximity, and ratings of 2 in touching (a and b), gazing, and affect. Descriptively, Michael always looked away from his mother's face, never vocalizing his need for her; he never reached toward or touched her and appeared intensely anguished and fearful. He frequently pulled away from touching her, did not relax when she held him, and rarely sought her out visually when she was apart from him. His mother rarely looked at him, never spoke to him, rarely touched him, and occasionally pulled away when he brushed against her. She held him stiffly and did not pick him up when he was distressed, occasionally leaving him to the pediatrician's care by going out of the room. Her affect was often unhappy and tense if not fearful.

The clinicians were concerned that Michael was suffering a preautistic condition and mobilized a program of intervention that combined surrogate parenting for the child and psychotherapy for the mother. As the therapeutic work progressed, it became clear that Michael's mother was a severely depressed woman who had experienced traumatic losses and physical abuse during her own childhood, alerting clinicians to the possibility that she might react with violence toward Michael (Helfer & Kempe, 1974). The mother's turning away during the pediatric examination was an ominous sign of how she might turn away from Michael at home during trying periods. Child abuse, which includes striking as well as neglecting a child, typically occurs when a parent is feeling threatened, abandoned, frightened, ungratified, or helpless—all responses to stressful events. If a parent is feeling desperate and an infant augments this with an additional demand (such as crying), the parent may decompensate behaviorally as well as emotionally. Michael was an unhappy-appearing infant who seemed little able to offer his mother spontaneous pleasure. These circumstances led those involved in the case to fear that Michael's mother might not be able to tolerate the strain of caring for her young child and might rid herself of Michael, who was indeed a burden to her; that she might isolate herself emotionally from Michael as well as from others; or that she might substitute a hallucinated or drug-induced alternative reality for her daily life.

The greatest therapeutic dividends for Michael's mother and for Michael derived from the mother's perception of her therapist's care; because she felt mothered she felt less deprived and was able to give more to her child. By the time Michael was sixteen months old, shifts on the Scale documented the increasing social involvement of mother and son, and it was evident that Michael was showing increasing pleasure in his contacts with people in general and in his adaptive, exploratory behavior in the environment.

## Conclusion

The value of the Scale lies in the promise of its utility for early detection and intervention in the service of the prevention of mental illness and disturbed development. Current research and clinical application of the scale will further understanding of its predictive capacity. Thus far, the scale has been useful in hospital and clinic settings in assisting in the early recognition of potentially disruptive patterns within parent-infant dyads. The scaled items are in a large measure a concise and coherent ordering of many of the theoretical and empirical assumptions upon which experienced infant mental health clinicians already base their therapeutic work.

To date the Scale has also shown itself to be effective in training clinicians to appreciate the range of interactions that normally occur between a mother and her infant. Not knowing precisely what is wrong with a parent and child, physicians-in-training have nonetheless been able to progress from the level of ambiguous comments such as, "Things just don't feel right with the case . . . the mother seems distant," to precise and replicable descriptions as they have familiarized themselves with Scale categories. As our experience with the children being followed progresses, we hope to publish additional reports. We also look forward to the reports of other investigators and practitioners who apply the ADS Scale as well as other measures of related early developmental phenomena.

The development of the Scale has received invaluable support from grants by the L. J. and Mary C. Skaggs Foundation, Oakland, California, and by many colleagues, chief among whom are Joe Afterman, Kathy Bacon, Abbot Bronstein, Justin Call, Linn Campbell, Eleanor Galenson, Martha Harris, Toni Heineman, Candy Pearce, Judith Rosenthal, Joel Saldinger, and Robert Zachary. Moses Grossman, Chief of Pediatrics at San Francisco General Hospital, and Richard Spates, Betty Tableman, and Mary K. Peterson of the Departments of Public Health and Mental Health of the State of Michigan have also offered critical assistance.

# References

Adelson, E. and Fraiberg, S. (1977). An abandoned mother, an abandoned baby. *Bulletin of the Menninger Clinic, 41,* 162–180.

Ainsworth, M., Blehar, M., Waters, E., and Wall, S. (1978). *Patterns of Attachment: A Psychological Study of the Strange Situation.* Hillsdale, New Jersey: Lawrence Erlbaum.

Bender, L. (1947). Childhood schizophrenia. *American Journal of Orthopsychiatry, 17,* 40–56.

Bowlby, J. (1951). *Maternal Care and Mental Health.* Geneva: World Health Organization.

Bowlby, J. (1969). *Attachment and Loss, vol. 1.* New York: Basic Books.

Brazelton, T. B. (1973). Neonatal behavioral assessment scale. *Clinics in Developmental Medicine, 50.* London: William Heinemann.

Call, J. (1963). Prevention of autism in a young infant in a well-child conference. *Journal of the American Academy of Child Psychiatry, 2,* 451–459.

Cameron, N. (1963). *Personality Development and Psychopathology.* Boston: Houghton Mifflin.

Campbell, B. K. (1977). An assessment of early mother-infant interaction and the subsequent development of the infant in the first two years of life. *Dissertation Abstracts International, 38.*

Christensen, M., Lee, C., and Bugg, P. (1979). Nurse practitioners as a function of need motivation, learning style, and locus of control. *Nursing Research, 28,* 51–60.

Condon, W. and Sander, L. (1974). Neonate movement is synchronized with adult speech. *Science, 83,* 99–101.

Early and Periodic Screening, Diagnosis and Treatment (EPSDT) Medicaid Program. (1969). Amended to the Social Security Act, Title XIX, Section 1905 (a).

Fantz, R. (1965). Visual perception from birth as shown by pattern selectivity. *New York Academy of Sciences, 118,* 793–814.

Fantz, R. and Miranda, S. (1975). Newborn infant attention to form of contour. *Child Development, 46,* 224–228.

Fraiberg, S., Adelson, E., and Shapiro, V. (1975). Ghosts in the nursery: A psychoanalytic approach to the problems of impaired infant-mother relationships. *Journal of the American Academy of Child Psychiatry, 14,* 387–421.

Freud, A. (1965). *Normality and Pathology in Childhood.* New York: International University Press.

Greenspan, S., Lourie, R., and Nover, R. (1979). A developmental approach to classification of psychopathology in infancy and early childhood. In *Basic Handbook of Child Psychiatry, vol. 2,* ed. J. Noshpitz. New York: Basic Books.

*Health, Education and Welfare (1975). Ambulatory Care Utilization Patterns of Children and Young Adults: National Ambulatory Medical Care Survey.* U.S. Department of Health, Education, Welfare, Vital and Health Statistics, Series 13, No. 39.

Helfer, R. and Kempe, C., eds. (1974). *The Battered Child.* Chicago: University of Chicago Press.

Hingtgen, J. and Bryson, C. (1972). Recent developments in the study of early childhood psychoses. *Schizophrenia Bulletin, 5,* 8–53.

Kanner, L. (1943). Autistic disturbances of affective contact. *Nervous Child, 2,* 217–250.

Kernberg, O. (1975). *Borderline Conditions and Pathological Narcissism.* New York: Jason Aronson.

Klaus, H. and Kennell, J. (1976). *Maternal-Infant Bonding: The Impact of Early Separation or Loss on Family Development.* St. Louis, Missouri: C. V. Mosby.

MacFarlane, J., Allen, L., and Honzik, M. (1962). *A Developmental Study of the Behavior Problems of Normal Children Between 21 Months and 14 Years.* Berkeley: University of California Press.

Mahler, M. and Furer, M. (1968). *On Human Symbiosis and the Vicissitudes of Individuation.* New York: International University Press.

Massie, H. (1975). The early natural history of childhood psychosis. *Journal of the American Academy of Child Psychiatry 14,* 683–707.

Massie, H. (1977). Patterns of mother-infant behavior and subsequent childhood psychosis. *Child Psychiatry and Human Development, 7,* 211–230.

Massie, H. (1978a). Blind ratings of mother-infant interaction in prepsychotic and normal infants. *American Journal of Psychiatry, 135,* 1371–1374.

Massie, H. (1978b). The early natural history of childhood psychosis: 10 cases studied by analysis of family home movies of the infancies of the children. *Journal of the American Academy of Child Psychiatry, 17,* 29–45.

Massie, H. (1979). Nonsystematic clinical observations of arterial oxygen saturation in newborns when held by the mother and nurses, which needs to be formally replicated. Unpublished.

Massie, H.(1980). Pathological interactions in infancy. In *High-Risk Infants and Children; Adult and Peer Interactions,* ed. T. Field et al. New York and London: Academic Press, 79–97.

National Institute of Mental Health. (1979). *Clinical Infant Intervention Research Programs.* Rockville, Maryland: United States Department of Health, Education and Welfare.

Ornitz, E. and Ritvo, E. (1976). The syndrome of autism. *American Journal of Psychiatry, 135,* 1371–1374.

Rank, B. (1955). Intensive study and treatment of preschool children who show marked personality deviations or "atypical development" and their parents. In *Emotional Problems of Early Childhood*, ed. G. Caplan. New York: Basic Books.

Roiphe, H. (1979). A theoretical overview of preoedipal development during the first 4 years of life. In *Basic Handbook of Child Psychiatry, vol. 1*, ed. J. Noshpitz. New York: Basic Books.

Rosenblith, J. (1979). The Graham/Rosenblith behavioral examination for newborns. In *Handbook of Infant Development*, ed. J. Osofsky. New York: Wiley.

Sameroff, A., ed. (1978). Organization and stability of newborn behavior: A commentary on the Brazelton Neonatal Behavior Assessment Scale. *Monograph Society for Research in Child Development, 43*.

Skinner, B. G. (1953). *Science and Human Behavior*. New York: MacMillan.

Sperling, M. (1974). *The Major Neuroses and Behavior Disorders in Children*. New York: Jason Aronson.

Spitz, R. (1965). *The First Year of Life*. New York: International University Press.

Spitz, R. and Wolf, K. (1946). The smiling response. *Genetic Psychology Monograph, 34*.

Stern, D. (1971). A micro-analysis of mother-infant interaction: Behavior regulating social contact between a mother and her 3½ month-old twins. *Journal of the American Academy of Child Psychiatry, 10*, 501–517.

Tronick, E., Als, H., Adamson, L., Wise, E., et al. (1978). The infant's response to entrapment between contradictory messages in face-to-face interaction. *Journal of the American Academy of Child Psychiatry, 17*, 1–13.

United States Department of Commerce (1977). *County and City Data Book*. Washington: United States Government Printing Office.

Watson, J. (1926). *Psychological Care of Infant and Child*. New York: Norton.

Willemson, E. (1977). Formulas developed in consultation with the Mother-Infant Development Project, Department of Psychology, University of Santa Clara, Santa Clara, California. Unpublished.

Winnicott, D. W. (1958). The capacity to be alone. In *The Maturational Processes and the Facilitating Environment*. New York: International Universities Press, 1965.

# Bibliography

Ainsworth, M. and Bell, S. Attachment, exploration, and separation: Illustration of one-year-olds in a strange situation. *Child Development*, 41:49–67, 1970.

Alexander, H. C. B. Insanity in children. *Journal of the American Medical Association*, 21:511–519, 1893.

Als, H., Tronick, B., and Brazelton, T. B., Affective reciprocity and the development of autonomy: the study of a blind infant. *Journal of the American Academy of Child Psychiatry*, 19:22–40, 1980.

American Psychiatric Association, Committee on Nomenclature and Statistics. *Diagnostic and Statistical Manual of Mental Disorders, Third Edition*. Washington, D.C.: American Psychiatric Association, 1980.

Anders, T. State and rhythmic process. *Journal of the American Academy of Child Psychiatry*, 17:224–238, 1978.

Andrew, R. J. The origin of facial expressions. *Scientific American*, 213:88–94, 1965.

Anthony, E. J. The significance of Jean Piaget for child psychiatry. *British Journal of Medical Psychology*, 19:20–34, 1956.

Anthony, E. J. An experimental approach to the psychopathology of childhood autism. *British Journal of Medical Psychology*, 32:211–225, 1958.

Anthony, E. J. The influence of maternal psychosis on children—folie à deux. In *Parenthood. Its Psychology and Psychopathology*. E. J. Anthony and T. Benedek (Eds.). Boston: Little, Brown and Company, 1970, 571–598.

Anthony, E. J. Naturalistic studies of disturbed families. In *Explorations in Child Psychiatry*, E. J. Anthony, (Ed.). New York: Plenum Press, 1975.

Anthony, E. J. The effects of abnormal parents on their infants and abnormal infants on their parents. Infant Psychiatry Symposium, Department of Psychiatry, University of California at San Francisco, November 14, 1980.

Arlow, J. Theories of pathogenesis. *Psychoanalytic Quarterly,* 50:488–514, 1981.

Bateson, G. et al. Toward a theory of schizophrenia. *Behavioral Science,* 1:251–264, 1956.

Bell, R. Q. A reinterpretation of the direction of effects in studies of socialization. *Psychological Review,* 75:81–95, 1968.

Bender, L. Childhood schizophrenia. *Nervous Child,* 1:138–140, 1942.

Bender, L. Childhood schizophrenia. *American Journal of Orthopsychiatry,* 17:40–56, 1947.

Bender, L. et al. A quantitative test of theory and diagnostic indicators of childhood schizophrenia. *American Medical Association Archives of Neurology and Psychiatry,* 70:413–427, 1953.

Bender, L. Twenty years of clinical research on schizophrenic children, with special reference to those under six years of age. In *Emotional Problems of Early Childhood.* New York: Basic Books, 1955.

Bender, L. Autism in children with mental deficiency. *American Journal of Mental Deficiency,* 64:81–86, 1959.

Bibring, G., et al. A study of the psychological processes in pregnancy and of the earliest mother-child relationship. *The Psychoanalytic Study of the Child,* 16:9–72. New York: Int. Univ. Press, 1961.

Birdwhistel, R. L. *Kinesics and Context.* Philadelphia: University of Pennsylvania Press, 1970.

Bleuler, E. Dementia Praecox or the Group of Schizophrenias. J. Zinkin (Tr.). New York: International Universities Press, 1911/1950.

Boatman, M. and Szurek, S. A clinical study of childhood schizophrenia. In *The Etiology of Schizophrenia.* D. Jackson (Ed.) New York: Basic Books, 1960.

Boismier, J. D. Visual stimulation and sleep-wakefulness behavior in the human newborn. Unpublished Ph.D. thesis, George Peabody College for Teachers, Nashville, Tennessee, 1973.

Bonnard, A. Primary process phenomena in the case of a borderline psychotic child. *The International Journal of Psychoanalysis,* 48:221–236, 1967.

Bower, T. G. The object in the world of the infant. *Scientific American,* 225:30–38, 1971.

Bowlby, J. The nature of the child's tie to his mother. *International Journal of Psychoanalysis,* 39:350–373, 1958.

Bowlby, J. *Attachment and Loss. Vol. 1. Attachment.* New York: Basic Books, 1969.

Bradley, C. *Schizophrenia in Childhood.* New York: Macmillan, 1941.

Brazelton, T. B. *The Neonatal Behavioral Assessment Scale.* Philadelphia: Lippincott, 1973.

Brazelton, T. B. and Als. H. Four early stages in the development of mother-infant interaction. *The Psychoanalytic Study of the Child.* 34:347–369. New Haven. Yale University Press, 1979.

Brazelton, T. B., Koslowski, B., and Main, M. The origins of reciprocity: the early mother-infant interaction. In Lewis, M. and Rosenblum, L. A. (Eds.). *The Effect of the Infant on Its Caregiver.* New York: Wiley, 1974, pp. 49–76.

Brazelton, T. B., Tronick, E., Adamson, L., Als, H., and Wise, W. Early mother-infant reciprocity. In *Parent-Infant Interaction.* Ciba Foundation Symposium, 33. New York: Associated Scientific Publishers, 1975, pp. 137–155.

Brody, S. *Patterns of Mothering.* New York: International Universities Press, 1956.

Brody, S. A mother is being beaten. In E. J. Anthony and T. Benedek (Eds.) *Parenthood: Its Psychology and Psychopathology.* Boston: Little, Brown, 1970.

Brody, S. and Axelrad, S. *Anxiety and Ego Formation in Infancy.* New York: International Universities Press, 1970.

Broucek, F. Efficacy in infancy. A review of some experimental studies and their possible implications for clinical theory. *International Journal of Psychoanalysis,* 60:311–316, 1979.

Brouzet, E. *Essai sur l'éducation médicinale des enfants et sur leurs maladies.* Paris, 1974.

Burrows, G. M. *Commentaries on the Causes, etc. of Insanity.* London, 1828.

Call, J. Newborn approach behavior and early social development. *International Journal of Psychoanalysis,* 45:286–294, 1964.

Call, J. and Marschak, M. Styles and games in infancy. *Journal of the American Academy of Child Psychiatry,* 5:193–210, 1969.

Campbell, S. and Taylor, P. Bonding and attachment: theoretical issues. *Seminars in Prenatology,* 3:3–13, 1979.

Cantwell, D. The diagnostic process and diagnostic classification in child psychiatry — *DSM-III* introduction. *Journal of the American Academy of Child Psychiatry,* 19:345–356, 1980.

Carpenter, G. C., Tecce, J., Stechler, G., and Friedman, S. Differential visual behavior to human and humanoid faces in early infancy. *Merrill-Palmer Quarterly of Behavior and Development,* 16:91–108, 1970.

Chappell, D. F. and Sander, L. W. Mutual regulation of the neonatal-maternal interactive process: context for the origins of communication. In *Before Speech: The Beginning of Interpersonal Communication.* M. Bullowa (Ed.). Cambridge: Cambridge University Press, 1979, pp. 89–109.

Chess, S., et al. Interaction of temperament and environment in the production of behavioral disturbances in children. *American Journal of Psychiatry,* 120:142, 1963.

Chess, S. Autism in children with congenital rubella. *Journal of Autism and Childhood Schizophrenia,* 4:33–41, 1974.

Chess, S. The plasticity of human development. *Journal of the American Academy of Child Psychiatry,* 17:80–91, 1978.

Chevalier-Skolnikoff, S. The ontogeny of primate intelligence and its implications for communicative potential. In *Origins and Evolution of Language and Speech.* S. Harnad, H. Stecklis, and J. Lancaster (Eds.). New York: New York Academy of Sciences, 1976.

Clevenger, S. V. Insanity in children. *American Journal of Neurology and Psychiatry,* 585–601, 1883.

Cohen, L. B., DeLoache, J., and Strauss, M. Infant visual perception. In *Handbook of Infant Development.* J. Osofsky (Ed.). New York: Wiley, 1979, pp. 393–438.

Condon, W. S. and Sander, L. W. Neonate movement is synchronized with adult speech: Interactional participation and language requisition. *Science:* 183:99–101, 1974.

Condon, W. S. Neonatal entrainment and enculturation. In Bullowa, M. (Ed.). *Before Speech. The Beginning of Interpersonal Communication.* Cambridge: Cambridge University Press, 1979, pp. 131–148.

Creak, M. Schizophrenic syndrome in childhood: report of a working party. *British Medical Journal,* 2:889–890, 1961.

Creak, M. Childhood psychosis: A review of 100 cases. *British Journal of Psychiatry*, 109:84–89, 1963.

Creak, M., et al. Clinical and EEG studies on a group of 35 psychotic children. *Developmental Medicine and Child Neurology*, 11:218–227, 1969.

Davis, H. A description of aspects of mother-infant vocal interaction. *Journal of Child Psychology and Psychiatry*, 19:379–386, 1978.

DeSanctis, S. On some varieties of dementia praecox. In *Clinical Studies in Childhood Psychosis*. S. A. Szurek and I. N. Berlin (Eds.). New York: Brunner/Mazel, 1973, pp. 31–47.

Despert, J. L. Thinking and motility disorder in schizophrenic child. *Psychiatric Quarterly*, 15:522–536, 1941.

Despert, J. L. Schizophrenia in children. *Psychiatric Quarterly*, 12:366–371, 1938.

Despert, J. L. *The Emotionally Disturbed Child — Then and Now*. New York: Vantage Press, 1965.

Diatkine, R., et al. Therapeutic experiences with psychotic children. In C. Chiland (Ed.). *Long-Term Treatment of Psychotic States*. New York: Human Sciences Press, 1977, pp. 250–258.

Eisenberg, L. Psychotic disorders in childhood. In *Biological Basis of Pediatric Practice*. R. E. Cook (Ed.). New York: McGraw-Hill, 1966.

Eisenberg, R. B. Auditory behavior in the human neonate. *International Audiology*, 8:34–45, 1969.

Ekstein, R. *Children of Time and Space of Action and Impulse. Clinical Studies on the Psychoanalytic Treatment of Severely Disturbed Children*. New York: Appleton–Century–Crofts, 1966.

Ekstein, R. and Caruth, E. Levels of verbal communication in the schizophrenic child's struggle against, for, and with the world of objects. *The Psychoanalytic Study of the Child*, 24:115–137. New York: International Universities Press, 1969.

Ekstein, R., Bryant, K., and Friedman, S. Childhood schizophrenia and allied conditions. In *Schizophrenia: A Review of the Syndrome*. L. Bellak (Ed.). New York: Logos Press, 1958, 555–693.

Emde, R. N., Gaensbauer, T. G., and Harmon, R. J., *Emotional Expression in Infancy: A Biobehavioral Study*. Psychological Issues, Monograph No. 37, Vol. 10. International Universities Press, 1976.

Emde, R. N. and Harmon, R. J. Endogenous and exogenous smiling systems in early infancy. *Journal of the American Academy of Child Psychiatry*, 11:177–200, 1972.

Emde, R. and Koenig, K. Neonatal smiling and rapid eye movement states. *Journal of the American Academy of Child Psychiatry*, 8:57–67, 1969.

Emde, R. N. and Robinson, J. The first two months: recent research in developmental psychobiology and the changing view of the newborn. In Call, J., Noshpitz, J., Cohen, R., and Berlin, I. (Eds). *Basic Handbook of Child Psychiatry, Vol. I, Development*. New York: Basic Books, 1979, 72–106.

Emde, R. and Walker, S. Longitudinal study of infant sleep: Results of 14 subjects studied at monthly intervals. *Psychophysiology*, 13:456–461, 1976.

Erikson, E. *Childhood and Society*. New York: W. W. Norton, 1950.

Esquirol, J. E. D. *Des Maladies Mentales*. Vol. I, Paris, 1838.

Fantz, R. L. The origin of form of perception. *Scientific American*, 204:66–72, 1961.

Fantz, R. L. Pattern vision in newborn infants. *Science*, 140:296–297, 1963.

Fantz, R. L. and Nevis, S. Pattern preferences and perceptual cognitive development in early infancy. *Merrill-Palmer Quarterly*, 13:77–108, 1967.

Fay, W. and Schuler, A. *Emerging Language in Autistic Children.* Baltimore: University Park Press, 1980.

Feldman, R. Therapeutic experiences with psychotic children. In. C. Chiland (Ed.). *Long-Term Treatment of Psychotic States.* New York: Human Sciences Press, 1977, pp. 258–265.

Ferber, A. Personal communication and film demonstration. Albert Einstein College of Medicine, 1972.

Field, T. Interaction patterns of high-risk and normal infants. In *Infants Born at Risk.* T. Field, A. Sostek, s. Goldberg, and H. Shuman (Eds.). New York: Spectrum, 1979.

Field, T. Infant gaze aversion and heart rate during face-to-face interactions. *Infant Behavior and Development,* 4:307–315, 1981.

Fish, B., et al. A classification of schizophrenic children under five years. *Am. J. of Psychiatry,* 124:1415–1423, 1968.

Fish, B. Biologic antecedents of psychosis in children. In Freedman, D. X. (Ed.). *The Biology of the Major Psychoses: A Comparative Analysis,* Vol. 54. New York: Raven Press, 1975, pp. 49–80.

Fish, B. An approach to prevention in infants at risk for schizophrenia: developmental deviations from birth to 10 years. *Journal of the American Academy of Child Psychiatry,* 15:62–82, 1976.

Fish, B. Neurobiologic antecedents of schizophrenia in children: evidence for an inherited, congenital and neurointegrative defect. *Archives of General Psychiatry,* 34:1297–1313, 1977.

Fish, B. The study of motor development in infancy and its relationship to psychological functioning. *Am. J. of Psychiatry,* 117:1113–1118, 1961.

Fish, B. The maturation of arousal and attention in the first months of life: A study of variations in ego development. *Journal of the American Academy of Child Psychiatry,* 2:253–270, 1963.

Fish, B. Longitudinal observations of biological deviations in a schizophrenic infant. *American Journal of Psychiatry,* 116:25–31, 1959.

Fish, B. and Ritvo, E. Psychoses of childhood. In *Basic Handbook of Child Psychiatry. Volume Two. Disturbances in Development.* J. Noshpitz (Ed.). New York: Basic Books, 1979.

Fish, B., et al. A typology of children's psychiatric disorders: I. Its application to a controlled evaluation of treatment. *Journal of the American Academy of Child Psychiatry,* 4:32–52, 1965.

Fraiberg, S. Smiling and stranger reaction in blind infants. In *The Exceptional Infant. Vol. 2. Studies in Abnormalities.* J. Hellmuth (Ed.). New York: Brunner/Mazel, 1971, pp. 110–127.

Fraiber, S. Pathological defense in infancy. Infant Psychiatry Symposium, Department of Psychiatry, University of California at San Francisco, May 1981.

Fraiberg, S. and Freedman, D. A. Studies in the ego development of the congenital blind child. *Psychoanalytic Study of the Child,* 19:133–169. New York: International Universities Press, 1968.

Freese, M. and Thoman, E. The assessment of maternal characteristics for the study of mother-infant interactions. *Infant Behavior and Development,* 1:95–105, 1978.

Freud, A. *The Ego and the Mechanisms of Defense. The Writings of Anna Freud. Vol. 2.* New York: International Universities Press (1937/1966).

Freud, A. *Normality and Pathology in Childhood: Assessments of Development. The Writings of Anna Freud. Vol. 6.* New York: International Universities Press, 1965.

Freud, A. Assessment of childhood disturbances. *The Psychoanalytic Study of the Child,* 17:149–158. New York: International Universities Press, 1962.

Freud, S. Three essays on the theory of sexuality. *Standard Edition, Vol. 6.* J. Strachey (Ed.). London: Hogarth Press, 1905/1955.

Freud, S. Instincts and their vicissitudes. *Standard Edition, Vol. 14.* J. Strachey (Ed.). London: Hogarth Press, 1915/1957.

Freud, S. The ego and the id. *Standard Edition, Vol. 19.* J. Strachey (Ed.). London: Hogarth Press, 1923/1961.

Freud, S. Inhibitions, symptons, and anxiety. *Standard Edition, Vol. 20.* J. Strachey (Ed.). London: Hogarth Press, 1926/1959.

Geleerd, E. R. A contribution to the problem of psychoses in childhood. *The Psychoanalytic Study of the Child,* 2:217–291. New York: International Universities Press, 1946.

Gellis, S. (Ed.). *Yearbook of Pediatrics.* Chicago: Yearbook Medical Publishers, 1974, pp. 313–315.

Goldfarb, W. Receptor preferences in schizophrenic children. *A.M.A. Archives of Neurological Psychiatry,* 76:643–652, 1956.

Goldfarb, W. *Childhood Schizophrenia.* Cambridge: Harvard University Press, 1961.

Goldfarb, W. An investigation of childhood schizophrenia. *Archives of General Psychiatry,* 11:620–634, 1964.

Goldfarb, W. Childhood psychosis. In *Carmichael's Manual of Child Psychology, Vol. II.* P. Mussen, (Ed.). New York: John Wiley and Sons, 1970, pp. 765–830.

Goldfarb, W., Meyers, D., Florsheim, J., Goldfarb, N. *Psychotic Children Grown Up.* New York: Human Sciences Press, 1978.

Gottfried, A. W. and Rose, S. Tactile recognition memory in infants. *Child Development,* 51:69–74, 1980.

Graham, P., Rutter, M., and George, S. Temperamental characteristics as predictors of behavior disorders in children. *American Journal of Orthopsychiatry,* 43:328–339, 1973.

Greding, J. E. Medical aphorisms on melancholy, etc. (1790). In *An Inquiry Into Mental Derangement II.* A. Crichton (Ed.). London, 1798.

Greenacre, P. The influence of infantile trauma on genetic patterns. In *Psychic Trauma.* S. S. Furst (Ed.). New York: Basic Books, 1967, pp. 108–153.

Greenacre. P. On focal symbiosis. In *Dynamic Psychopathology in Childhood.* L. Jessner and E. Pavenstadt (Eds.). New York: Grune and Stratton, 1959, pp. 243–256.

Greenacre, P. Toward an understanding of the physical nucleus of some defense reactions. *International Journal of Psychoanalysis,* 39:69–76, 1958.

Greenacre, P. Pregenital patterning. *International Journal of Psychoanalysis,* 33:410–415, 1952.

Greenman, G. W. Visual behavior of newborn infants. In Solnit, A., and Provence, S. (Eds.). *Modern Perspectives in Child Development.* New York: International Universities Press, 1963.

Greenspan, S. I. *Intelligence and Adaptation. An Integration of Psychoanalytic and Piagetian Developmental Psychology.* New York: International Universities Press, 1979.

Haith, M. Visual scanning in infants. In Stone, L. J., Smith, H. T., and Murphy, L. B. (Eds.). *The Competent Infant: A Handbook of Readings.* New York: Basic Books, 1973, pp. 320–323.

Haith, M. Visual competence in early infancy. In Herd, R., Leibowitz, H., and Teuber, H. L. (Eds.). *Handbook of Sensory Physiology, VIII.* New York: Springer, 1976.

Haith, M. *Rules That Babies Look By. The Organization of Newborn Visual Activity.* Hillsdale: Lawrence Erlbaum Associates, 1980.

Haith, M. and Campos, J. Human infancy. *Annual Review of Psychology*, 28:251–293, 1977.

Harlow, H. and Harlow, M. Effects of various mother-infant relationships on Rhesus monkey behaviors. In *Determinants of Infant Behavior, Vol. 14.* B. M. Foss (Ed.). London: Methuen, 1956.

Harmon, R. J., et al. Infants' preferential response for mother vs. an unfamiliar adult: relationship to attachment. *Journal of American Academy of Child Psychiatry*, 18:437–450, 1979.

Hartmann, H. *Ego Psychology and the Problem of Adaptation.* New York: International Universities Press, 1958.

Hartmann, H., Kris, E., and Loewenstein, R. Comments on the formation of psychic structure. *The Psychoanalytic Study of the Child*, 11:11–38. New York: International Universities Press, 1947.

Haslam, J. *Observations on Madness.* 2nd Edition. London, 1809, pp. 185–206.

Haynes, H., White, B., and Held, R. Visual accommodation in human infants. *Science*, 148:528–530, 1965.

Heller, T. About dementia infantalis. W. C. Hulse (tr.). *Journal of Nervous and Mental Disorders*, 119:471–477, 1930/1954.

Hellmuth, J. (Ed.). *Exceptional Infant, Volume 1. The Normal Infant.* New York: Brunner/Mazel, 1967.

Hellmuth, J. (Ed.). *Exceptional Infant. Studies in Abnormalities. Volume 2.* New York: Brunner/Mazel, 1971.

Henshenson, M. Visual discrimination in the human newborn. *Journal of Comparative and Physiological Psychology*, 58:270–276, 1964.

Hershenson, M. Development of the perception of form. *Psychological Bulletin*, 67:326–336, 1967.

Hingtgen, J. and Bryson, C. Recent developments in the study of early childhood psychoses. *Schizophrenia Bulletin*, 5:8–53, 1972.

Hutt, S. J., Lenard, H. C., and Prechtel, H. Psychophysiological studies in newborn infants. In Lipsitt, L. and Reese, H. (Eds.). *Advances in Child Development and Behavior, Vol. 4.* New York: Academic Press, 1969, pp. 127–172.

Kazan, J. and Lewis, M. Studies of attention in the human infant. *Merrill-Palmer Quarterly*, 11:95–127, 1965.

Kagan, J., et al. Infants' differential reactions to familiar and distorted faces. *Child Development*, 37:519–532, 1966.

Kanner, L. Problems of nosology and psychodynamics of early infantile autism. *American Journal of Orthopsychiatry*, 19:416–426, 1949.

Kanner, L. To what extent is early infantile autism determined by constitutional inadequacies? *Genetics and the Inheritance of Integrated Neurological Psychiatric Patterns. Research Publications of the Association for Research in Nervous and Mental Disease*, 33:378–385, 1953.

Kanner, L. Childhood psychosis: A historical overview. *Journal of Autism and Childhood Schizophrenia*, 1:14–19, 1971.

Kanner, L. *Child Psychiatry, Fourth Edition* (1972). Springfield, Illinois: Charles Thomas, 1935.

Kanner, L. Autistic disturbances of affective contact. *Nervous Child*, 2:217–250, 1943.

Kanner, L. Early infantile autism. *Journal of Pediatrics*, 25:211–217, 1944.

Kanner, L. Irrelevant and metaphorical language in early infantile autism. *American Journal of Psychiatry*, 103:242–246, 1946.

Kasinin, J. and Kaufman, M. R. A study of the functional psychoses in childhood. *American Journal of Psychiatry,* 86: 307–384, 1929.

Kaufman, B. *Son Rise.* New York: Warner Books, 1976.

Kendon, A. Some functions of gaze direction in social interaction. *Acta Psychologica,* 26:22–63, 1967.

Kennell, J. H. et al. The effect of early mother-infant separation on later maternal performance. *Pedatric Research,* 4:473–474, 1970.

Kennell, J. H. et al. Maternal behavior one year after early and extended post-partum contact. *Developmental Medicine and Child Neurology,* 16:172–179, 1974.

Kennell, J. and Klaus, M. Early mother-infant contact: effects on the mother and the infant. *Bulletin of the Menninger Clinic,* 43:69–78, 1979.

Kerlin, I. N. Juvenile insanity. *Transactions of the Medical Society of Pennsylvania,* 12:611–620, 1879.

Kernberg, O. *Object Relations Theory and Clinical Psychoanalysis.* New York: Jason Aronson, 1976.

Kernberg, P. Childhood psychosis: A psychoanalytic perspective. In S. Greenspan and G. Pollock (Eds.). *The Course of Life, Psychoanalytic Contributions Toward Understanding Personality Development. Volume I: Infancy and Early Childhood.* Washington: National Institute of Mental Health, 1980, pp. 603–617.

Kety, S., et al. The types and prevalence of mental illness in the biological and adoptive families of adopted schizophrenics. In Rosenthal, D. and Kety, S. (Eds.). *The Transmission of Schizophrenia.* Oxford: Pergamon Press, 1968, pp. 345–362.

Klaus, M. H., et al. Maternal attachment: importance of the first post-partum days. *New England Journal of Medicine,* 286:460–463, 1972.

Klein, M. *Contributions to Psychoanalysis 1921–1945.* London: Hogarth Press, 1948.

Klein, M. On Mahler's autistic and symbiotic phases. An exposition and evaluation. *Psychoanalysis and Contemporary Thought. A Quarterly of Integrative and Interdisciplinary Studies,* 4:69–106, 1981.

Knobloch, H. and Pasamanick, B. Some etiologic and prognostic factors in early infantile autism and psychosis. *Pediatrics,* 55:182–191, 1975.

Kohut, H. *The Analysis of the Self. A Systematic Approach to the Psychoanalytic Treatment of Narcissistic Personality Disorders.* New York: International Universities Press, 1971.

Korner, A. and Thoman, E. Visual alertness in neonates as evoked by maternal care. *Journal of Experimental Child Psychology,* 10:67–78, 1970.

Kraeplin, E. *Dementia Praecox and Paraphrenia.* Chicago: Chicago Medical Book, 1919.

Lewis, M. Infants' responses to facial stimuli during the first year of life. *Developmental Psychology,* 1:75–86, 1969.

Lewis, M., and Goldberg, S. Perceptual-cognitive development in infancy. A generalized expectancy model as a function of the mother-infant interaction. *Merrill-Palmer Quarterly,* 15:81–100, 1969.

Lewis, M. and Rosenblum, L. (Eds.). *The Effect of the Infant on its Caregiver.* New York: Wiley, 1974.

Loewald, H. Instinct theory, object relations and psychic structure formation. *Journal of the American Psychoanalytic Association,* 26:493–506, 1978.

Lutz, J. Uber die Schizophrenie im kindesalter. *Schweiz. Archives Neurological Psychiatry,* 39:335–372, 1937.

MacDonald, J. Insanity in a healthy boy, four years old. *New York Journal of Medicine,* 8–9, 1846.

McCall, R. B., Hagerty, P. S., Hamilton, J. S. and Vincent, J. M. Habituation rate and the infant's response to visual discrepancies. *Child Development,* 44:280–287, 1973.

McCall, R. B. and Kagan, J. Stimulus schema discrepancy and attention in the infant. *Journal of Experimental and Child Psychology*, 5:381–390, 1967.

Mahler, M. S. On childhood psychosis and schizophrenia: autistic and infantile psychoses. *Psychoanalytic Study of the Child*, 7:286–306, 1952.

Mahler, M. S. Autism and symbiosis: two extreme disturbances of identity. *Int. J. Psychoanalysis*, 39:77–83, 1958.

Mahler, M. S. *On Human Symbiosis and the Vicissitudes of Individuation. Vol. I. Infantile Psychosis.* New York: International Universities Press, 1968.

Mahler, M., Ross, J. R. and DeFries, Z. Clinical studies in benign and malignant cases of childhood psychosis. *American Journal of Orthopsychiatry*, 19:295–305, 1949.

Mahler, M. S. and Gosliner, B. J. On symbiotic child psychosis. *The Psychoanalytic Study of the Child*, 10:195–215, 1955.

Mahler, M. S., Furer, M. and Settlage, C. F. Severe Emotional Disturbances in Childhood: Psychosis. In *American Handbook of Psychiatry, Volume One*. S. Arieti (Ed.). New York: Basic Books, 1959, pp. 816–839.

Mahler, M. S. and Furer, M. Child psychosis: a theoretical statement and its implications. *Journal of Autism and Childhood Schizophrenia*, 2:213–218, 1972.

Mahler, M. S. and McDevitt, J. B. Observations on adaptation and defense in stati nascendi. *Psychoanalytic Quarterly*, 37:1–22, 1968.

Mahler, M., Pine, F., and Bergman, A. *The Psychological Birth of the Human Infant.* New York: International Universities Press, 1975.

Mahler, M. Longitudinal study of the treatment of a psychotic child with the tripartite design. In *The Selected Papers of Margaret Mahler. Volume I. Infantile Psychosis and Early Contributions.* New York: Jason Aronson, 1976/1979, pp. 233–261.

Mahler, M. On early infantile psychosis: the symbiotic and autistic syndromes. *Journal of the American Academy of Child Psychiatry*, 4:554–568, 1965.

Mahler, M. On sadness and grief in infancy and childhood: Loss and restoration of the symbiotic love object. *The Psychoanalytic Study of the child*, 16:332–351. New York: International Universities Press, 1961.

Massie, H. The early natural history of childhood psychosis. *Journal of the American Academy of Child Psychiatry*, 14:683–707, 1975.

Massie, H. Patterns of mother-infant behavior and subsequent childhood psychosis: A research and case report. *Child Psychiatry and Human Development*, 7:211–230, 1977.

Massie, H. The early natural history of childhood psychosis: 10 cases studied by analysis of family home movies of the infancies of the children. *Journal of the American Academy of Child Psychiatry*, 17:29–45, 1978.

Massie, H. Blind ratings of mother-infant interaction in prepsychotic and normal infants. *American Journal of Psychiatry*, 135:1371–1374, 1978.

Massie, H. and Campbell, B. K. The Scale of Mother-Infant Attachment Indicators During Stress (AIDS Scale). In Call, J., Galenson, E., Tyson, R. (Eds.). *Frontiers of Infant Psychiatry*. New York: Basic Books, 1983, pp. 394–412.

Maudsley, H. *Physiology and Pathology of Mind.* London: 1880.

Meltzhoff, A. and Moore, M. Imitations of facial and manual gestures by human neonates. *Science* 198:75–78, 1977.

Mercurialis, H. De Morbis Puerorum (1583). Quoted in Ruhrah, J. *Pediatrics of the Past.* New York, 1925.

Meyers, D. and Goldfarb, W. Psychiatric appraisals of parents and siblings of schizophrenic children. *American Journal of Psychiatry*, 118:902–908, 1962.

Mises, R., et al. Essai d'approche psychopathologique de la déficience intellectuelle: les déficits dysharmoniques. *Psychiatrie enfant*, 14:341–464, 1971.

Morison, T. C. Case of mania in a child six years old. *Journal of Psychological Medicine*, 1:317, 1948.

Ornitz, E. and Ritvo, E. The syndrome of autism: a critical review. *American Journal of Psychiatry*, 133:609–621, 1976.

Paine, R. S., et al. *Neurological Examination of Children*. London: Spastics Society, 1966.

Parmalee, A. and Stern, E. Development of states in infants. In Clemente, C. D., Purpura, D. P., and Mayer, F. E. (Eds.). *Sleep and the Maturing Nervous System*. New York: Academic Press, 1972, pp. 199–228.

Perfect, W. *Annals of Insanity*. 2nd Edition. London, 1801, pp. 251–281.

Philips, I. Discussion of E. J. Anthony's paper "The Infants of Depressed Mothers." Infant Psychiatry Symposium, Department of Psychiatry, University of California at San Francisco, November 14, 1980.

Piaget, J. *The Origins of Intelligence in Children*, M. Cook, (Tr.). New York: International Universities Press, 1937/1952.

Piaget, J. *The Construction of Reality in the Child*, M. Cook (Tr.). New York: Basic Books, 1936/1954.

Pines, D. Pregnancy and motherhood: interaction between fantasy and reality. *British Journal of Medical Psychology*, 45:333–343, 1972.

Potter, H. W. Schizophrenia in children. *American Journal of Psychiatry*, 89:1253–1270, 1933.

Prechtl, H. F. The behavioural states of the newborn infant (a review). *Brain Research*, 76:185–212, 1974.

Prechtl, H. F. and Beintema, D. *The Neurological Examination of the Full-Term Newborn Infant*. London: Heinemann, 1964.

Rank, B. and Macnaughton, D. A clinical contribution to early ego development. *The Psychoanalytic Study of the Child*, 5:53–65, New York: International Universities Press, 1950.

Rank, B. Intensive study and treatment of preschool children who show marked personality deviations, or "atypical development," and their parents. In *Emotional Problems of Early Childhood*. G. Caplan (Ed.). New York: Basic Books, 1955, 491–502.

Richmond, W. The dementia praecox child. *American Journal of Psychiatry*, 88:1153–1159, 1932.

Rimland, B. The syndrome and its implication for a neural theory of behavior. *Infantile Autism*. New York: Appleton-Century-Crofts, 1964.

Robson, K. The role of eye-to-eye contact in maternal infant attachment. *Journal of Child Psychology and Psychiatry*, 8:13–25, 1967.

Robson, K. and Moss, H. Patterns and determinants of maternal attachment. *Journal of Pediatrics*, 77:976–985, 1970.

Roffwarg, H. P., Muzio, J. N., and Dement, W. C. Ontogenetic development of the human sleep-dream cycle. *Science*, 152:604–619, 1966.

Rosenthal, J., Massie, H., and Wulff, K. A comparison of cognitive development in normal and psychotic children in the first two years of life from home movies. *Journal of Autism and Developmental Disorders*, 10:433–444, 1980.

Rubenstein, E. A. Childhood mental disease in America. A review of the literature. *American Journal of Orthopsychiatry*, 18:314–321, 1948.

Rush, B. *Medical Inquiries and Observations Upon Diseases of the Mind*. Philadelphia, 1812, pp. 56–57.

Rutter, M. Behavioral and cognitive characteristics of a series of psychotic children. *Childhood Autism: Clinical, Educational and Social Aspects*. J. K. Wong (Ed.). London: Pergammon Press, 1966.

Rutter, M. Psychological development: Predictions from infancy. *Journal of Child Psychiatry and Psychology,* 11:49–62, 1970.

Rutter, M. *Maternal Deprivation Re-assessed.* Middlesex: Penguin Books, 1978.

Rutter, M. The development of infantile autism. *Psychological Medicine,* 4:147–163, 1974.

Rutter, M. Individual differences. In Rutter, M. and Hersov, L. (Eds.). *Child Psychiatry: Modern Approaches.* London: Blackwell Scientific Publications, 1977.

Rutter, M., Birch, H. G., and Chess, S. Temperamental characteristics in infancy and the later development of behavioral disorders. *British Journal of Psychiatry,* 110:651–661, 1964.

Rutter, M. and Lockyear, L. A five- to fifteen-year follow-up study of infantile psychosis. I: Description of the sample. *British Journal of Psychiatry,* 113:1169–1182, 1967.

Rycroft, C. *A Critical Dictionary of Psychoanalysis.* New York: Basic Books, 1968.

Sameroff, A. J. and Chandler, M. J. Reproductive risk and the continuum of caretaking casualty. In *Review of Child Development Research. Vol. 4.* F. D. Horowitz, et al. (Eds.). Chicago: University of Chicago Press, 1975.

Sander, L. Infant and caretaking environment: investigation and conceptualization of adaptive behavior in a system of increasing complexity. In Anthony, E. J. (Ed.), *Explorations in Child Psychiatry,* 129–166. New York: Plenum Press, 1975.

Sander, L. and Julia, H. continuous interactional monitoring in the neonate. *Psychosomatic Medicine,* 28:822–835, 1966.

Schaffer, H. R., Collis, G. M., & Parsons, G. Vocal interchange and visual regard in verbal and preverbal children. In *Studies in Mother-Infant Interaction.* London: Academic Press, 1977.

Scheflen, A. *Body Language and Social Order.* Englewood Cliffs, N.J.: Prentice-Hall, 1972.

Seguin, E. *Traitement Moral des Idiots.* Paris, 1846.

Shafii, M. Childhood Psychosis. In J. Noshpitz (Ed.), *Basic Handbook of Child Psychiatry, Vol. 3.* New York: Basic Books, 1979, pp. 555–567.

Spitz, R. A. Anxiety in infancy: A study of its manifestations in the first year of life. *International Journal of Psycholanalysis,* 31:138–143, 1950.

Spitz, R. The primal cavity: a contribution to the genesis of perception and its role for psychoanalytic theory. *The Psychoanalytic Study of the child,* 10:215–240. New York: International Universities Press, 1955.

Spitz, R. The derailment of dialogue, stimulus overload, action cycles, and the completion gradient. *Journal of the American Psychoanalytic Association,* 12:752–775, 1964.

Spitz, R. *A Genetic Field Theory of Ego Formation: Its Implication for Pathology.* New York: International Universities Press, 1959.

Spitz, R. *The First Year of Life.* New York: International Universities Press, 1965.

Spitz, R., Emde, R. N., and Metcalf, D. R. Further prototypes of ego formation: A working paper from a research project on early development. *The Psychoanalytic Study of the Child,* 5:417–441. New York: International Universities Press, 1970.

Spitzka, E. C. *Insanity, Its Classification, Diagnosis and Treatment.* Birmingham, 1883.

Sroufe, L. Alan and Waters, E. The ontogenesis of smiling and laughter: a perspective on the organization of development in infancy. *Psychological Review,* 83:173–189, 1976.

Stechler, G. and Latz, E. Some observations on attention and arousal in the human neonate. *Journal of the American Academy of Child Psychiatry,* 5:517–525, 1966.

Sterman, M. B. The basic rest-activity cycle and sleep. In *Sleep and the Maturing Nervous*

*System.* C. B. Clemente, D. P. Purpura, and F. E. Mayer (Eds.). New York: Academic Press, 1972.

Stern, D. A micro-analysis of mother-infant interaction: behavior regulating social contact between a mother and her 3½-month old twins. *Journal of the American Academy of Child Psychiatry,* 10:501–517, 1971.

Stern, D. The goal and structure of mother-infant play. *Journal of the American Academy of Child Psychiatry,* 13:402–412, 1974.

Stern, D. Mother and infant at play. In *The Effect of the Infant on the Caregiver,* M. Lewis and L. Rosenblum (Eds.). New York: Wiley, 1974, pp. 187–213.

Stern, D., et al. Vocalizing in unison and in alternation: two modes of communication within the mother-infant dyad. *Annals of the New York Academy of Science,* 263:89–100, 1975.

Stern, D., Jaffe, J., Beebe, B., and Bennett, S. Vocalizing in unison and in alternation. *Transactions of New York Academy of Science, Conference on Developmental Linguistics and Communication Disorders,* 1975.

Stone, L. J., Smith, H. T., and Murphy, L. B. (Eds.). *The Competent Infant. Research and Commentary.* New York: Basic Books, Inc., Publishers, 1973.

Szurek, S. Childhood schizophrenia: Psychotic episodes and psychotic maldevelopment. *American Journal of Orthopsychiatry,* 26:519–543, 1956.

Szurek, S. Attachment and psychotic detachment. In S. Szurek and I. A. Berlin (Eds.). *Clinical Studies in Childhood Psychosis.* New York: Brunner/Mazel, 1973, pp. 191–277.

Taylor, J. M. The insane disorders of childhood. *Archives of Pediatrics,* 11:100–115, 1894.

Thomas, A., Chess, S., and Birch, H. *Temperament and Behavior Disorders in Children.* New York: University Press, 1968.

Thomas, H. Visual fixation responses of infants to stimuli of varying complexity. *Child Development,* 36:629–638, 1965.

Thomas, R., et al. Comments on some aspects of self and object representation in a group of psychotic children. *The Psychoanalytic Study of the Child,* 21:527–580. New York: International Universities Press, 1966.

Tolpin, M. On the beginnings of a cohesive self: an application of the concept of transmuting internalization to the study of the transitional object and signal anxiety. *The Psychoanalytic Study of the Child,* 26:316–354. New York: Quadrangle Books, 1972.

Torrey, E. F., Hersh, S. P., and McCabe, K. D. Early childhood psychosis and bleeding during pregnancy. A prospective study of gravid women and their offspring. *Journal of Autism and Childhood Schizophrenia,* 5:287–297, 1966.

Trevarthen, C. Primary intersubjectivity. In Schaffer (Ed.). *Studies in the Mother-Child Interaction.* New York: Academic Press, 1978.

Tronick, E., Als, H., Adamson, L., Wise, S., Brazelton, T. B. The infant's response to entrapment between contradictory messages in face-to-face interaction. *Journal of the American Academy of Child Psychiatry,* 7:1–13, 1978.

Voisin, F. *Des Causes Morales et Physiques des Maladies Mentales.* Paris, 1926.

Walk, A. The prehistory of child psychiatry. *British Journal of Psychiatry,* 110:754–767, 1964.

Watson, J. S. Smiling, cooing, and the yawns. *Merrill Palmer Quarterly of Behavior Development,* 18:323–340, 1972.

Weil, A. P. Clinical data and dynamic considerations in certain cases of childhood schizophrenia. *American Journal of Orthopsychiatry,* 23:518–529.

Werry, J. Childhood psychoses. In H. C. Quay and J. Werry (Eds.). *Psychopathological Disorders of Childhood.* New York: John Wiley, 1972.

White, B. L., Castle, P. and Held, R. Observations on the development of visually-directed reaching. *Child Development,* 35:349–364, 1969.

Winnicott, D. W. *Mother and Child. A Primer of First Relationships.* New York: Basic Books, 1957.

Winnicott, D. W. *The Maturational Process and the Facilitating Environment.* New York: International Universities Press, 1965.

Witmer, L. What I did with Don. In S. A. Szurek and I. A. Berlin (Eds.). *Clinical Studies in Childhood Psychosis.* New York: Brunner/Mazel, 1919/1973, pp. 48–64.

Witmer, L. Orthogenic cases XIV, Don: A curable case of arrested development due to fear psychosis and the result of shock in a three-year-old infant. *Psychology Clinic,* 13:97–111, 1919–1922.

Wolf, K. and Spitz, R. Anaclitic depression. An inquiry into the genesis of psychiatric conditions in early childhood, II. *The Psychoanalytic Study of the Child,* 2:312–342. New York: International Universities Press, 1946.

Wolff, P. The developmental psychologies of Jean Piaget and Psychoanalysis. *Psychological Issues,* Monograph No. 5. New York: International Universities Press, 1960.

Wolff, P. Observations on the early development of smiling. In Foss, B. (Ed.). *Determinants of Infant Behavior,* 2:113–134, New York: Wiley, 1963.

Wolff, P. The development of attention in young infants. *Annals of the New York Academy of Science,* 118:815–830, 1965.

Wolff, P. The causes, controls and organization of behavior in the neonate. *Psychological Issues,* Monograph No. 17, New York: International Universities Press, 1966.

Wolff, P. The natural history of crying and other vocalizations in early infancy. In Foss, B. (Ed.). *Determinants of Infant Behavior,* 4:81–109, 1969, London: Methuen.

Wolff, P. and White, B. L. Visual pursuit and attention in young infants. *Journal of the American Academy of Child Psychiatry,* 4:473–484, 1965.

Wynne, L. and Singer, M. Thought disorder in family relations of schizophrenics. *Archives of General Psychiatry,* 9:191–198, 1963.

# Index

Accessory symptoms, 12
  *(See also specific accessory symptoms, for example:* Hallucinations)
Activity level and activities, 14
  of autistic children, 100, 101, 103, 104, 108, 113, 132
  and basic rest-activity cycle, 53
  low, as defense behavior, 219
  of symbiotic psychotic children, 120, 130, 132
  *(See also* Hyperactivity)
Acute fulmination, insidious-onset childhood schizophrenia followed by, 13
Acute-onset childhood schizophrenia, 13
Acute symptoms, 248–250
  behavior modification for life-threatening, 248, 250
  drugs for, 249, 250
  *(See also specific acute symptoms, for example:* Self-aggression)
Adelson, E., 270
Administration of ADS Scale, 267–268
ADS Scale *(see* Massie-Campbell Scale of Mother-Infant Attachment Indicators During Stress)
Adult psychiatry, development of child psychiatry influenced by, 11, 13
Adult schizophrenia, 1, 2, 13–14, 21, 22, 28, 231
Advanced defense mechanisms, 218, 219

Affect, 4, 228
  of autistic children, 104, 105, 112–114, 130, 132, 139, 142
  as defined in ADS Scale, 265
  isolation of, 219
  in mixed form of early childhood psychosis, 133
  of prepsychotic and normal infants, compared, 153, 157, 161, 162
  of symbiotic psychotic children, 126, 127
Affective consummation:
  failures of, 212–213, 228
  impediments to, 183–184
Affective development, 56–59
  and affective capacity for object constancy, 167
Affective disorders, 9, 12, 28
  *(See also* Depression)
Afterman, J., 280
Age-appropriate behaviors of normal and prepsychotic children, compared, 170–172, 178
Age of onset, 16, 26, 37
  of autism, 20
  of childhood schizophrenia, 13, 20, 28
  delusions and hallucinations and, 37
  DSM-III classification and, 28
  of later childhood psychosis, 30
  of manic-depressive psychosis, 28

## About the Authors

**Henry N. Massie,** M.D., is Director of Child Psychiatry Residency Training at McAuley Neuropsychiatric Institute, St. Mary's Hospital, San Francisco, California, and Assistant Clinical Professor of Psychiatry at the University of California School of Medicine, San Francisco. Dr. Massie received his child psychiatry training at Mt. Zion Hospital in San Francisco and his advanced training at the San Francisco Psychoanalytic Institute. He is the author of numerous articles in the field of normal child development and in clinical child and adult psychiatry. Dr. Massie also maintains a private practice in child and adult psychiatry in San Francisco.

**Judith Rosenthal,** M.S.W., is a developmental psychologist and a clinical social worker. She is Research Associate in the Study of the Second Year of Life at the San Francisco Psychoanalytic Institute.